Medicine and Colonial Identity

Individuals or groups define their identities in particular ways, choosing from a long list of social variables: nationality, class, race, gender, age, sexuality, occupation, or marital status, all of which may change, either by choice, or fate. Over the last century, the issue of identity has become increasingly important, and yet it remains a problematic category of historical analysis.

The historical record is full of diplomats and peasants discussing medicine and health concerns and topics which are significant to the study of medicine – professionalization, therapeutic choice, medical education, and medical practice – topics which allow us to juxtapose a number of different strands of identity. This volume shows how the study of medicine can provide new insights into colonial identity, and serves as a means to accommodate multiple perspectives on identity within a single narrative. An international range of contributors explore a variety of issues including:

- the perceived self-identity of colonizers
- the adoption of Western and traditional medicine as complementary aspects of a new, modern, and nationalist identity
- the creation of a modern identity of women in the colonies
- the expression of a healer's identity by physicians of traditional medicine

Medicine and Colonial Identity will be of essential interest to those studying the history of medicine and will also be of value to social historians.

Mary P. Sutphen is currently completing a book entitled *Imperial Hygiene: Medicine and Public Health in the British Empire, 1880–1931*, an analysis of the history of laboratory medicine in the British Empire. **Bridie Andrews** is an Associate Professor at Harvard University. Her publications include *The Making of Modern Chinese Medicine* and an edited volume with Andrew Cunningham entitled *Western Medicine as Contested Knowledge*.

Routledge studies in the social history of medicine
Edited by Bernard Harris, *University of Southampton*, Joseph Melling, *University of Exeter* and Anne Borsay, *University of Wales at Lampeter*

The Society for the Social History of Medicine was founded in 1969, and exists to promote research into all aspects of the field, without regard to limitations of either time or place. In addition to this book series, the Society also organises a regular programme of conferences, and publishes an internationally-recognised journal, *Social History of Medicine*. The Society offers a range of benefits, including reduced-price admission to conferences and discounts on SSHM books, to its members. Individuals wishing to learn more about the Society are invited to contact the series editors through the publisher.

The Society took the decision to launch 'Studies in the Social History of Medicine', in association with Routledge, in 1989, in order to provide an outlet for some of the latest research in the field. Since that time, the series has expanded significantly under a number of series editors, and now includes both edited collections and monographs. Individuals wishing to submit proposals are invited to contact the series editor in the first instance.

1. **Nutrition in Britain**
Science, scientists and politics in the twentieth century
Edited by David F. Smith

2. **Migrant, Minorities and Health**
Historical and contemporary studies
Edited by Lara Marks and Michael Worboys

3. **From Idiocy to Mental Deficiency**
Historical perspectives on people with learning disabilities
Edited by David Wright and Anne Digby

4. **Midwives, Society and Childbirth**
Debates and controversies in the modern period
Edited by Hilary Marland and Anne Marie Rafferty

5. **Illness and Healing Alternatives in Western Europe**
Edited by Marijke Gijswit-Hofstra, Hilary Marland and Has de Waardt

6. **Health Care and Poor Relief in Protestant Europe 1500–1700**
Edited by Ole Peter Grell and Andrew Cunningham

7. **The Locus of Care**
Families, communities, institutions, and the provision of welfare since antiquity
Edited by Peregrine Horden and Richard Smith

8. **Race, Science and Medicine, 1700–1960**
Edited by Waltraud Ernst and Bernard Harris

9. **Insanity, Institutions and Society, 1800–1914**
Edited by Bill Forsythe and Joseph Melling

10. **Food, Science, Policy and Regulation in the Twentieth Century**
International and comparative perspectives
Edited by David F. Smith and Jim Phillips

11. **Sex, Sin and Suffering**
Venereal disease and European society since 1870
Edited by David F. Smith and Jim Phillips

12. **The Spanish Influenza Pandemic of 1918–1919**
New perspectives
Edited by Howard Phillips and David Killingray

13. **Plural Medicine, Tradition and Modernity, 1800–2000**
Edited by Waltraud Ernst

14. **Innovations in Health and Medicine**
Diffusion and resistance in the twentieth century
Edited by Jenny Stanton

15. **Contagion**
Historical and cultural studies
Edited by Alison Bashford and Claire Hooker

16. **Medicine, Health and the Public Sphere in Britain, 1600–2000**
Edited by Steve Sturdy

17. **Medicine and Colonial Identity**
Edited by Mary P. Sutphen and Bridie Andrews

18. **New Directions in the History of Nursing**
Edited by Barbara E. Mortimer and Susan McGann

Medicine and Colonial Identity

Edited by Mary P. Sutphen
and Bridie Andrews

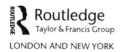

LONDON AND NEW YORK

First published 2003
by Routledge
2 Park Square, Milton Park, Abingdon, Oxfordshire OX14 4RN

Simultaneously published in the USA and Canada
by Routledge
711 Third Avenue, New York, NY 10017

First issued in paperback 2015

Routledge is an imprint of the Taylor and Francis Group, an informa business

© 2003 Editorial matter and selection, Mary P. Sutphen and Bridie Andrews, individual chapters, the contributors

Typeset in Sabon by
BOOK NOW Ltd

All rights reserved. No part of this book may be reprinted or reproduced or utilised in any form or by any electronic, mechanical, or other means, now known or hereafter invented, including photocopying and recording, or in any information storage or retrieval system, without permission in writing from the publishers.

British Library Cataloguing in Publication Data
A catalogue record for this book is available from the British Library

Library of Congress Cataloging in Publication Data
Medicine and colonial identity / edited by Mary P. Sutphen and Bridie Andrews.
　　p. cm.
　　Includes bibliographical references and index.
　　1. Medicine–History. 2. Colonialism. 3. Identity (Psychology) 4. Colonies–Health aspects. I. Sutphen, Mary P., 1960– II. Andrews, Bridie.

R133 .M3696 2003
610′.9–dc21
　　　　　　　　　　　　　　　　　　　　　　　　　　　　　　　　　　2002031930

ISBN 13: 978-1-138-86793-2 (pbk)
ISBN 13: 978-0-415-28880-4 (hbk)

Contents

	List of contributors	ix
	Acknowledgments	xi
1	Introduction BRIDIE ANDREWS AND MARY P. SUTPHEN	1
2	"The ignorance of women is the house of illness": gender, nationalism, and health reform in colonial north India MANEESHA LAL	14
3	A sword of empire?: medicine and colonialism at King William's Town, Xhosaland, 1856–91 DAVID GORDON	41
4	Midwives, missions and reform: colonizing Dutch childbirth services at home and abroad *ca.* 1900 HILARY MARLAND	61
5	New Zealand milk for 'building Britons' PHILIPPA MEIN SMITH	79
6	Tropical medicine and colonial identity in northern Australia SUZANNE PARRY	103
7	Colonial doctors and national myths: on telling lives in Australian medical biography ROY MACLEOD	125
	Index	143

Contributors

Bridie Andrews is an Associate Professor at Harvard University. Her publications include *The Making of Modern Chinese Medicine* (Cambridge University Press, forthcoming), and she has previously edited a volume with Andrew Cunningham entitled *Western Medicine as Contested Knowledge* (Manchester University Press, 1997).

David Gordon's research interests include environmental change, culture and politics in the history of central and southern Africa. He is Assistant Professor of History at the University of Maryland College Park and teaches pre-colonial and modern African history. He has authored several scholarly articles on topics in south and central African history and is preparing a manuscript on history and eco-politics in a central African fishery.

Maneesha Lal received her Ph.D. from the Department of History and Sociology of Science at the University of Pennsylvania and has taught at Penn and the University of Wisconsin, Madison. She held a post-doctoral research fellowship from the Ministère de l'Education Nationale in France and is currently at the Columbia University Institute for Scholars at Reid Hall in Paris. She is completing a manuscript on the history of women physicians in colonial India.

Roy MacLeod is Professor of History at the Universitiy of Sydney. He was educated at Harvard, the London School of Economics and Cambridge, and has held senior positions at the Universities of Sussex and London, and visiting appointments in Paris, Amsterdam, Oxford, and the University of California (Santa Cruz). He has taught and written extensively in the history of science and medicine in Britain, and on science and medicine in the expansion of Europe.

Hilary Marland is Senior Lecturer in History and Director of the Centre for the History of Medicine at the University of Warwick. She is former editor of *Social History of Medicine*, and has published on midwifery and childbirth in the Netherlands, nineteenth-century medical practice in England, women and medicine, and infant and maternal welfare. She is currently working on puerperal insanity in nineteenth-century Britain and preparing a monograph study, *Dangerous Motherhood: Insanity and Childbirth in the Nineteenth Century*.

Phillippa Mein Smith is Senior Lecturer in History at the University of Canterbury, Christchurch, New Zealand, and is an overseas member of the editorial board of *Social History of Medicine*. Her publications include *Maternity in Dispute: New Zealand 1920–1939* (Wellington: Historical Branch, 1986), *Mothers and King Baby: Infant Survival and Welfare in an Imperial World: Australia 1880–1950* (London: Macmillan, 1997), and Donald Denoon and Philippa Mein Smith, with Marivic Wyndham, *A History of Australia, New Zealand and the Pacific* in the Blackwell History of the World series (Oxford: Blackwell, 2000)

Suzanne Parry is a Senior Lecturer at the Northern Territory University in northern Australia. She is currently researching the history of leprosy in Australia, having published an earlier work on the Channel Island Leprosarium. She has also published on the health of indigenous people in northern Australia in colonial and postcolonial times.

Mary P. Sutphen is completing a manuscript entitled "Imperial Hygiene: Medicine and Public Health in the British Empire, 1880–1931" that analyzes the history of laboratory medicine in the British Empire.

Acknowledgments

This volume began in Oxford in 1996, when the Society for the Social History of Medicine (SSHM) hosted the conference, "Medicine and the Colonies." The co-organizers, Harriet Deacon and Molly Sutphen, tried to bring together participants from all over the world to debate the state of colonial medical history. One theme that surfaced in a number of papers was how different actors defined their colonial identities, and this volume was born.

When Harriet, who had worked indefatigably on the conference and on the early stages of this volume, needed to step aside, Bridie Andrews graciously took her place. We are very grateful to Harriet for her hard work, her intellectual rigor, and her tact.

We are indebted to Bernard Harris for his careful reading of the entire manuscript, sound editorial advice, and faith in this project. Special thanks are due to Poornima Sardesai, who contributed to the project from the beginning, and whose chapter would have been a valuable addition to this collection. Two anonymous reviewers gave us valuable suggestions for our introduction. We would also like to thank Peter Buck for his sharp and adroit comments on the introduction. Finally we thank Joe Whiting for his patience.

We gratefully acknowledge the Wellcome Trust, which provided financial support to the "Medicine and the Colonies" Conference in Oxford and to Bridie Andrews, Harriet Deacon, and Molly Sutphen.

Chapter 3 by David Gordon originally appeared as "A sword of empire? Medicine and colonialism in colonial Xhosaland," in *African Studies*, 60: 2 (2001), pp. 165–83 (http://www.tandf.co.uk).

1 Introduction

Bridie Andrews and Mary P. Sutphen

This volume examines aspects of medicine in relation to the articulation of identity in colonial settings. All of the chapters were presented at the 1996 "Medicine and the Colonies" Conference which the Society for the Social History of Medicine (SSHM) hosted in Oxford. At that conference, we were struck by the ways in which the study of medicine repeatedly threw up new insights on aspects of identity. There were papers on the perceived self-identity of colonizers (something represented here by David Gordon (Chapter 3), Hilary Marland (Chapter 4), Suzanne Parry (Chapter 6), and Roy MacLeod (Chapter 7)) while others highlighted the adoption of Western *and* traditional medicine as complementary aspects of a new, modern, and nationalist identity (represented here by Maneesha Lal (Chapter 2)). The creation of a modern identity for women in the colonies (Lal (Chapter 2) and Marland (Chapter 4)) was another aspect, as was the expression of a healer's identity by physicians of traditional medicine (Gordon (Chapter 3)).

Over the last century, identity as an avenue of inquiry has become an academic growth industry. There are two issues bound up in this: one is the distinctly Western notion of the discrete, bounded self; the Cartesian self which, in Michel Foucault's words, "places its own point of view at the origin of all historicity [and] which, in short, leads to a transcendental consciousness."[1] This individual identity has been the subject of extensive study since Freud and the rise of psychoanalytic theory in the early twentieth century. The second issue is group or collective identity, and the processes of *identification* by which people sort their environment into like and unlike, self and other. It is identity in this second sense which has generated so much recent scholarly attention from historians, sociologists, and anthropologists, and with which we are mainly concerned.

Feminist scholars have been carving out new fields in the study and critique of gendered identities in modern societies since the mid-twentieth century.[2] Much literature, both feminist and otherwise, has drawn on Foucault's work to emphasize corporeal aspects of identity: the body as the substrate upon which particular aspects of identity are performed.[3] In both of these trends, the interplay between individual and group identities has served to problematize categories of identity: as elsewhere in scholarship, much emphasis has been on heterogeneity, hybridity, and difference.

Recent work on nationalism as the dominant modern form of collective identity has led to a spirited debate on its relationship to colonialism. The dissolution of the Soviet Union after 1989 and the subsequent resurgence of national and ethnic identities, often with violent consequences, has given this debate special urgency.[4] In colonial history, an important part of daily life for colonial subjects was coming to terms with the identity labels that colonists applied to them. This became evident in 1997 during the debates over how many residents of British Hong Kong could be "awarded" full British citizenship before Hong Kong was returned to the People's Republic of China in 1997. In the early twentieth century, leaders of nationalist movements in the colonies claimed the right to local self-definition (today we might say "self-determination") as a crucial part of their agendas. This applied at the local level as much as at the national: for example, women identified as "female laborers" by colonial observers might have described themselves very differently. Instead of "workers", they were just as likely to think of themselves in kinship terms: as daughters-in-law, wives, and mothers. The negotiation of other people's identity labels was constitutive of colonial society long before it became the integral aspect of modern life that it is today.

Twenty-odd years ago, several historians of India proposed the study of a group they dubbed *subalterns*, both as a correction to the metropolitan focus of most colonial historiography, and also as creative response to Foucault's emphasis on the discourses of power and Antonio Gramsci's investigations of the mechanisms of political hegemony.[5] In 1981, when the *Subaltern Studies* collective began to publish, they privileged the experiences of these non-élite, aiming to resurrect local identities from the silence of the existing, élitist historiography. They were motivated to demonstrate how subjective identity, local concerns and the unseen workings of the imperial order could be used to explain Indian history from the bottom up. The founding editor of Subaltern Studies, Ranajit Guha, claimed that "subordination cannot be understood except as one of the constitutive terms in a binary relationship of which the other is dominance."[6] Without limiting themselves to a single defining identity of colonial subjectivity, subalternist historians have tended to make the praxis of rebellion the primary focus of their inquiries. Problematically, however, few sources survive in which the subalterns of Subaltern Studies expressed themselves directly. An apparently bipolar and one-dimensional relationship between dominant imperialists and subaltern subjects is exaggerated by the fact that many of the sources for subaltern history published to date are the same as those of the old imperial history. That is, although the Subaltern Studies collective aimed to undermine the view from the metropolis, it has been restricted by the relative abundance of sources in the archives of the colonial powers. They may be able to read these sources "against the grain," but the range of subjects that can be explored in this way has been determined in advance by the nature of the imperial collections. Gayatri Spivak cites Ranajit Guha's manifesto for recovering subaltern agency despite this lack:

> It is of course true that the reports, despatches, minutes, judgements, laws, letters, etc. in which policemen, soldiers, bureaucrats, landlords, usurers and others hostile to insurgency register their sentiments, amount to a representation of their will. But these documents do not get their content from that will alone, for the latter is predicated on another will – that of the insurgent. It should be possible therefore to read the presence of a rebel consciousness as a necessary and pervasive element within that body of evidence.[7]

Reading sources against the grain allows historians to discuss the agency of subjects who left behind no archival sources of their own: people otherwise without a history. Yet this agency, or will, is – according to Spivak – no more than a subject-effect. The effect of insurgency demands a "continuous and homogenous cause for this effect, and thus posits a sovereign and determining subject."[8] As she maintains in a later article, the subaltern – this posited, homogenized subject – cannot speak.[9]

Yet the category of "subaltern classes" is one which Guha himself acknowledges to include, "*ideally speaking* [emphasis in original] the lowest strata of the rural gentry, impoverished landlords, rich peasants and upper-middle peasants."[10] It would be surprising if all of these historical subalterns turned out to have been illiterate and to have left no written records at all. In fact there were many Indian newspapers in various vernacular languages, starting as early as 1810, and published in substantial numbers by the 1830s and '40s. It is hard to say why these and other vernacular sources have received so little attention in the rewriting of Indian history "from the bottom up." Much of the early vernacular literature was published under religious auspices of various kinds: some newspapers in local languages were funded by foreign missionaries; others were published in Urdu for a Muslim readership; and still other Indian-run papers displayed a Hindu religiosity far removed from the secular Hindu nationalism that modern scholarship is comfortable with. The historical interplay of religious issues with the development of insurgency towards colonial rule and the growth of nationalism is a particularly thorny field in the context of modern India. We suggest, however, that there are more subaltern voices in the historical record than are often acknowledged. In the field of medical history, a recent article by Deepak Kumar demonstrates how the use of sources in Telugu, Tamil, Malayalam, and Kannada as well as Hindi and English may shed useful new light on the interplay of Western and indigenous medicine from the point of view of "subaltern" medical practitioners.[11]

The inability to speak in an unmediated way is by no means confined to the subalterns of colonial history. In 1986, a group of anthropologists aired their discomfort with the relationship between anthropologists as authors and the subjects of anthropology, their "informants."[12] Contributors to a volume devoted to the debate questioned the representation of foreign cultures by students who were in the process of building careers for themselves; they doubted the reliability of informants when so many narrated their culture in return for an exchange of money, gifts, or social capital; and they indicated that the act of "giving voice" to previously silent peoples was in itself patronizing, if not also imperialist. In the soul-searching that followed what was dubbed the "Clifford and Marcus" debate, it seemed that all representations of "others" were hopelessly tainted, undermining the entire project of ethnography.

The "Clifford and Marcus" debate was, in part, a response to the writings of Edward Said. In *Orientalism*, Said drew on Michel Foucault's development of the notion of a discourse that is the extension and expression of a power relation to describe western writings on the East. "In brief," he wrote, "because of Orientalism the Orient was not (and is not) a free subject of thought or action." And: "European culture gained in strength and identity by setting itself off against the Orient as a sort of surrogate and even underground self."[13] As James Clifford noted in his introduction to the volume, Said documented the creation of a coherent "Orient" from multiple sources, a creation which "confer[ed] on the other a discrete entity, while also providing the knowing observer with a standpoint from which to see without being seen, to read without interruption."[14]

The undermining of this standpoint, this "place of overview" was the aim of the authors of the volume, but to the degree that they were successful, it left scholars in a quandary. As George Marcus put it: how can ethnography "define its object of study in ways that permit detailed, local, contextual analysis and simultaneously the portrayal of global implicating forces?"[15] To translate this problematic into the terms of our project, the crass lumping of colonial subjects by an imperial power and the local subjectivity of individuals are two ends of the spectrum of perceived identity. At the one end we find historians writing studies where diplomats play the starring roles, and at the other end, we find others trying to coax rebellious subalterns to speak more loudly.[16] Perhaps these two disjunctures are less serious than Marcus suggests: in studying local cultures, we often find that global forces are turned to unexpected ends. Detailed field study makes possible new understandings of the transnational context. This is true of several of the studies presented here.

Identity, then, is a kind of cultural commodity, important as a political or economic asset. While individuals or groups define their identities in particular ways, government officials, researchers, neighbors, or television reporters may impose different labels. They may choose from a long list of social variables: nationality, class, race, gender, age, sexuality, occupation, or marital status, all of which may change, either by choice or fiat. Thus a wife who kills her husband after a violent disagreement may be regarded as a murderess, as a victim of domestic abuse, or simply as a widow. The advantages to the woman of claiming the identity of victim may make the difference between life imprisonment or immediate freedom. Clearly, all ascriptions of identity status depend upon the context of the observer and the subject; they are open to multiple interpretations; and they are negotiable.

For all of these reasons, identity is a problematic category of historical analysis. Even when silences in the historical record do not force historians to focus on one aspect of identity, in practice it is still very difficult to write history that does justice to more than a couple of strands of identity. Should region trump class, and sex trump religion? Our understanding of these categories is in itself a modern phenomenon, and as outlined above, controversies over their importance are recent and rarely integral to the historical record. Scholarly studies reify the separation of particular strands of identity, as we can see in the thorough Manchester University Press series, History and Related Disciplines: Select Bibliographies, where one of the recent volumes organizes studies under the apparently exclusive headings of race, *or* gender, *or* religion, etc.[17] Other volumes are devoted entirely to a single characterizing identity.[18]

One way to get around this dearth of independent source materials is to look for topics that open up new windows on colonial existence. We suggest that medicine may provide a means to accommodate multiple perspectives within a single narrative. Although rarely talking with each other, the historical record is full of diplomats and peasants discussing medicine and health concerns. To pursue a metaphor, we use medicine as a shuttle to traverse the many strands of identity and attempt to weave an account that has the potential to reconcile a number of perspectives. The topics we cover in medicine – professionalization, therapeutic choice, medical education, and medical practice – allow us to juxtapose a number of strands of identity, without privileging one or two.

Other historians of medicine have done this to good effect, as we can see in a recent example on American medicine by Judith Leavitt.[19] She demonstrates that for American doctors, medicine has often been only one aspect of their identity as breadwinners. A day's work for nineteenth-century doctors might involve as much farming, trading, and child-care as it did medicine. As fathers or mothers, wives or husbands, businessmen and women, many doctors practiced medicine in a variety of settings – their own homes or in other people's – and within a large economic web. We found this study of doctors in their day-to-day rounds useful in its illumination of medical identity outside of the territory that historians have traversed so often in their discussions of professionalization.

We are, of course, not the first to notice how usefully the study of medical issues can illuminate aspects of social history. The literature on the medicine of empires is already rich.[20] In focusing on medicine and identity, we argue that the contributors to this volume inflect previous scholarship on the "medical pluralism" of many colonial situations with new meaning.[21] The idea of "pluralism" in medicine has been used to describe situations in ideologically neutral terms. A new clinic opens and people quickly learn how its services can benefit them, given their existing health-seeking behavior patterns. Resembling the rational choice model of economic behavior, studies of medical pluralism often interpret the health-seeking behavior of colonial subjects as based on their assessments of medical efficacy and social and monetary cost. The studies collected here argue that medicine can also be a key aspect of the cultural positioning by which colonists and colonized alike defined both themselves and the colonial other.

The sociologist Stuart Hall has argued that identity is an inherently unstable concept: that we construct our identities discursively by appropriating representations which acquire meaning from their contrast with other, different accounts. "Identities", he writes, "are about questions of using the resources of history, language and culture in the process of becoming rather than being; not 'who we are' or 'where we came from', so much as what we might become, how we have been represented and how that bears on how we might represent ourselves."[22] In culturally heterogenous situations, identities are constructed from the interwoven strands of multiple discourses and strategies. In this volume, medicine appears as one such category of discourse. It is deployed as a strategy of representation, and often one which historical actors have used to suture different aspects of their own identities. Through these medical fragments, we are contributing to a growing body of work which attempts to avoid the grand narratives – and indeed the grand counter-narratives – of colonial history, preferring instead to emphasize local stories of specific, named actors in their efforts to turn changing circumstances to best practicable advantage. The resulting picture of contingency and hybridity in the constitution of colonial identities will, we hope, help make the "others" of colonial history seem less foreign, and make visible the historical actors' most pressing concerns in their own terms.

We start in India with a study of gender, nationalism, and health reform in colonial North India, in which Maneesha Lal (Chapter 2) re-examines several aspects of the received wisdom about the process by which women and men acquired an Indian nationalist sense of identity under British rule. Her lens is the influential Hindi women's journal *Stri Darpan* [The Mirror of Women], founded in 1909 by Rameshwari Nehru, an aristocratic woman who had married into the influential Nehru clan. Lal finds that preoccupations with health-maintenance and hygiene in the pages of *Stri Darpan* were just as likely to look to Ayurvedic ideas of health management – now included under the new, umbrella concept of "hygiene" – as to Western medical knowledge. This attention by the upper-caste, middle-class to Ayurveda was part of the nationalist agenda, dedicated to promoting a proper appreciation of India's cultural heritage.

Stri Darpan also published many articles about the role of women in the modernizing Indian state, emphasizing education for women, especially in subjects essential to the rearing of healthy young citizens: nutrition, hygiene, and physical education. A range of opinions was published concerning the proper place of women in society, but all agreed on women's essential role.

Interestingly, Lal finds that the authors of many of these pedagogical articles were men, often licentiates of the Indian Medical Service (IMS). Not only this, but the various colonial initiatives to bring Western medicine, hygiene and education to Indian women (such as the Countess of Dufferin Fund) were rarely mentioned. Woman physicians, whether British or Indian, rarely appear. The inevitable conclusion is that the search for "a medical and healing theory and practice that was at once authentically 'Indian', yet 'modern'" was first and foremost a nationalist project, to which changes to Indian women's and medical identities were necessary, but subsidiary projects.

David Gordon's "A sword of empire? Medicine and colonialism at King William's Town, Xhosaland, 1856–91" (Chapter 3) examines the relationship between Europeans and Africans through a contextualized examination of the records of one British doctor, John Patrick Fitzgerald. Unlike the other chapters that focus on a collective identity, Gordon examines an individual who lived in rural South Africa for many years. The trade-off with such a biographical focus is the difficulty in drawing general conclusions, but we are richly rewarded with a rare glimpse of how one colonial doctor did and did not change his practices in the face of local pressures and colonial policy. In 1856, Fitzgerald was appointed head of the Medical Department of British Kaffraria and Superintendent of Native Hospitals, and was in charge of the King William's Town hospital until 1891. This appointment had been made by Sir George Grey, Governor of the Cape from 1854 to 1861, in the hope that the Western hospital would "transfer responsibility for healing from the rebellious and powerful African healers, . . . to a corps of European or European-trained doctors loyal to imperial authority." What Gordon demonstrates is that far from achieving this transfer of responsibility and authority, the Xhosa healers were able to assimilate Fitzgerald and his foreign healing practices into their own medical worldviews. An essential part of the Xhosa healing process was for patients to "assent" to their illness and to study the arts of healing from the practitioner, both to effect a cure and to become apprentice healers themselves. Fitzgerald's records indicate that it was not unusual for Xhosa healers to bring their own afflictions to him, to assent to his diagnosis and prescribed therapy, and to remain at the hospital for sometimes quite extended periods in order to learn the foreign ways of healing. For his part, Fitzgerald maintained a conviction of the value of teaching Western medicine to African students long after this ceased to be colonial policy. He demonstrated a willingness to learn from his African colleagues that was common in colonial situations in the first half of the nineteenth century, but became increasingly rare as Western medicine became more technologically sophisticated, and African and other indigenous healers were seen as less of a threat.

Gordon draws two important conclusions from his study: first, that colonial medicine could become part of local therapeutic cultures without destroying indigenous cultural identities or spreading colonial hegemony. Second, he observes that as Western medicine became part of the progressive science of the late nineteenth century, modernity came to be measured in contrast to the "traditionalism," "backwardness," and "savagery" of indigenous cultures. With the rise of modernity, white South Africans found it increasingly difficult to imagine any constructive engagement with indigenous cultures.

For the most part, the chapters in this volume focus on the British Empire, but we have also included a chapter that does not fall into this traditional configuration, but where the structure of the relationship between two regions exhibit features of colonialism. Hilary Marland's chapter (Chapter 4) studies the social movements to provide modern midwifery to both the southern provinces of the Netherlands and the Dutch East Indies in the late nineteenth and early twentieth centuries. In both cases, the Dutch central government was motivated to demonstrate its ability to provide modern health care. The fact that governments felt responsible for providing adequate medical facilities was new in the mid-nineteenth century, and medical reform was one of the ways that states established their credentials as modern and civilized.[23] But there was more than state and national identity at stake in the attempts to bring modern midwifery to the Roman Catholic southern provinces: the mainly Protestant northerners saw it as a duty to try to "civilize" their poorer, Catholic compatriots, while wealthy Catholics were inspired to protect "Catholic womanhood." This aspect of religious identity resulted in the recruitment of Catholic young women from poorer regions with the intention that they should return home once trained. In both the Dutch East Indies and in the southern provinces at home, reform activists drew attention to the "dangerous" and "superstitious" traditional practices associated with childbirth. And in both cases, the very fact of having received a midwifery education changed the identity of the students, who found it difficult to maintain practices in the poor, rural districts they had been trained for. By far the majority of those trained ended up in the more prosperous towns and developed areas, both at home and in the Dutch colonies. In both cases, the values embedded in attempts to extend state medical provision were intended to encourage a particular version of national identity.

In her account of how milk became associated with the healing and health of the body politic, Mein Smith (Chapter 5) pulls together imperial, national, gender, and racial strands of New Zealand identity, and we see them as a whole. From World War I, when New Zealand came to be one of the main suppliers of dairy products to Britain, until 1973, when Britain entered the European Economic Community (now the European Union), dairy farmers, nutritionists, eugenicists, school doctors, and experts on children made milk what Mein Smith called a "cultural icon" that was central to the image of

New Zealand as a clean, healthy, and green nation. New Zealand's dependence on British markets, medical arguments, and the maternal and child welfare programs and other social experiments that New Zealand was willing to undertake made milk into a commodity that mothers in Britain and the empire could count on to ensure a strong, healthy race. The production and consumption of milk would allow New Zealand and Britain to produce strong, robust, and white children to populate the British empire. During the 1930s, milk came to be seen as crucial in schools to the creation of healthy citizens, and the state supplied milk to all school children. The school milk programs also came into being just after the Depression, just at a point when dairy farmers most needed state support. World War II reinvigorated New Zealand's efforts to define their imperial identity, and Mein Smith found once again close ties between British imperial identity and milk. In a case study on milk in Christchurch in the 1950s, debates over whether to pasteurize milk surfaced, with those who advocated raw milk considering their cause as a way of "fighting to preserve . . . freedom and the British way of life." After the 1960s, when Britain entered what is now the European Union and the relationship between New Zealand and Britain changed, so too did the identity of milk. Mein Smith shows how men came to be the target of milk marketing, and the fluid so long associated with the message that children needed the drink to be strong, loyal citizens of empire, became a man's drink, one that would increase their strength and productivity.

In "Tropical medicine and colonial identity in northern Australia," Suzanne Parry (Chapter 6) describes how medical concerns were central to the establishment of a separate white colonial identity in the remote northern regions of Australia. The Australian government perceived it necessary for white Australians to inhabit all parts of the Australian landmass, as protection against immigration from Asia. However, at the turn of the twentieth century it was far from clear that white settlers could survive in the tropical northern territories. An Institute of Tropical Medicine was established in the north in 1911 to investigate questions of quarantine, endemic disease, and physiological responses to the climate. Although it was quickly established that none of these issues was a real hindrance to white settlement, tropical medicine soon became an instrument of internal colonialism. Northern settlers were outnumbered by the aboriginal population, and defined their own identity as northerners in contrast both to this population and to the more "civilized" south. Medical issues became the key measures of the backwardness of the Aborigines: not only were they untutored in the basics of the new sanitary science from Europe, but they were also catastrophically susceptible to a whole host of infectious diseases from the same source. Where outbreaks of infectious diseases might be mild or easily controlled among the (partially immune) white settlers, the aboriginal communities developed virulent epidemics. These spread rapidly beyond the purview of the colonial authorities, and threatened to re-infect white society. Ironically, while the diseases were being introduced by white settlers and

Chinese migrant labor, and spread through social and sexual intercourse at the fringes of aboriginal and settler society, it was the aboriginal sick who bore the brunt of colonial medical policing. Parry gives several vivid examples of how aboriginal identity, as a political force as well as a cultural one, has many of its roots in responses to the imposition of such medically-justified oppressions as enforced exclusion, detention, and relocation to native reservations.

In "Colonial doctors and national myths," Roy MacLeod (Chapter 7) takes the successive volumes of the *Australian Dictionary of Biography* and subjects the entries on medical practitioners to scrutiny. In this, he is concerned both with what the entries can tell us about the lives of colonial doctors, and what we may conclude about the concerns of the authors of these biographies: what, historically, have been the attitudes of those responsible for reducing an individual's identity to a dictionary entry? Perhaps inevitably, in the latter category, he finds Australian values to be attached only to white males, a trend that is only slowly showing signs of change. In the earliest period, to 1790, most medical entries refer to men who came as assistant naval surgeons, alongside a smaller number of medically-trained transported convicts. Like the American physicians described by Judith Leavitt, most nineteenth-century Australian physicians were also active in other fields, typically farming, business, or politics. Their identities were complex, therefore, and modern studies of their activities in terms of "professionalization" are anachronistic. The *ADB* entries also emphasize the values of self-reliance, survival skills in the face of adversity, and virtuous demise central to the creation of an Australian frontier identity.

In conclusion, we note that in a recent study of responses to malaria in Zimbabwe, JoAnn McGregor and Terence Ranger concluded that their investigations of local ideas and debates revealed "understandings of bodily health as part of a broad set of relationships between individuals, community, state and the land."[24] This volume is an attempt to further demonstrate how investigations of medical ideas, behavior, ideology and practice may shed new light on the construction of colonial identities.

Notes

1. Michel Foucault, *The Order of Things: An Archaeology of the Human Sciences*. London: Routledge, 1994, p. xiv.
2. A necessarily partial selection from this huge literature – selected for relevance to identity issues – includes Simone de Beauvoir, *The Second Sex*. Trans. and ed. H. M. Parshley. New York: Random House, 1974; Kate Millett, *Sexual Politics*. New York: Avon, 1969; Germaine Greer, *The Female Eunuch*. London: MacGibbon & Kee, 1970; Juliet Mitchell, *Psychoanalysis and Feminism*. New York: Pantheon, 1974; Carol Gilligan, *In a Different Voice: Psychological Theory and Women's Development*. Cambridge: Harvard University Press, 1982; Angela Davis, *Women, Race and Class*. New York: Random House, 1981; Donna Haraway, "A Manifesto for Cyborgs: Science, Technology, and Socialist

Feminism in the 1980s." *Socialist Review* (80 1985): 65–108; Joan W. Scott, "Gender: A Useful Category of Historical Analysis." *American Historical Review* (91 1986): 1053–75; Deborah K. King, "Multiple Jeopardy, Multiple Consciousness: The Context of a Black Feminist Ideology." *Signs* 14 (1 1988): 42–72; Chantal Mouffe, "Feminism, Citizenship, and Radical Democratic Politics." In Judith Butler and Joan W. Scott (eds), *Feminists Theorize the Political*. New York: Routledge, 1992: 369–84; Judith Butler, *Gender Trouble: Feminism and the Subversion of Identity*. New York: Routledge, 1990.
3 An excellent study of the importance of bodies as a site of colonialism is E. M. Collingham, *Imperial Bodies*. Cambridge: Polity Press, 2001.
4 Ernest Gellner's work was a touchstone in the development of this literature, for example in *Nations and Nationalism*. Ithaca: Cornell University Press, 1983. See also Elie Kedourie (ed.), *Nationalism in Asia and Africa*. New York: Meridian, 1970; Benedict Anderson, *Imagined Communities. Reflections on the Origin and Spread of Nationalism*. Revised edn, London and New York: Verso, 1991; C. A. Bayly, *Origins of Nationality in South Asia*. Delhi: Oxford University Press, 1998; Partha Chatterjee, *Nationalist Thought and the Colonial World – a Derivative Discourse?* London: Zed Books for the United Nations University, 1986; Eric Hobsbawm, *Nations and Nationalism since 1780: Programme, Myth, Reality*. Cambridge: Cambridge University Press, 1990; Kathryn A. Manzo, *Creating Boundaries: The Politics of Race and Nation*. Boulder: Lynne Rienner, 1996; Sumit Sarkar, *Writing Social History*. Delhi: Oxford University Press, 1997, esp. ch. 9, "Identity and Difference."
5 The Subaltern Studies collective was established to investigate South Asian history, though historians from other regions have developed similar perspectives. From the Subaltern Studies collective, see for example, Ranajit Guha and Gayarti Chakrvorty Spivak, *Selected Subaltern Studies*. Oxford: Oxford University Press, 1988, or Ranajit Guha, *Elementary Aspects of Peasant Insurgency in Colonial India*. Delhi: Oxford University Press, 1983. For similar perspectives, see James C. Scott and Benedict J. Tria Kerkvliet (eds), *Everyday Forms of Peasant Resistance in South-East Asia*. London : Frank Cass, 1986.
6 Ranajit Guha, "Preface," in *Selected Subaltern Studies*, p. 35.
7 Ranjit Guha, *Elementary Aspects of Peasant Insurgency in Colonial India*. Delhi: Oxford University Press, 1983, p. 15. Cited by Spivak in her Introduction (p. 13) to *Selected Subaltern Studies*. For a searching critique of the Subaltern Studies project, see Rosalind O'Hanlon, "Recovering the Subject: *Subaltern Studies* and Histories of Resistance in Colonial South Asia." *Modern Asian Studies* (22, 1 1988): 189–224.
8 Spivak, Introduction in *Selected Subaltern Studies*, p. 4
9 Gayatri Chakravorty Spivak, "Can the Subaltern Speak?" In Cary Nelson and Lawrence Grossberg (eds), *Marxism and the Interpretation of Culture*. London: Macmillan, 1988.
10 Guha, *Elementary Aspects*, p. 44.
11 Deepak Kumar, "Unequal Contenders, Uneven Ground: Medical Encounters in British India, 1820–1920." In Andrew Cunningham and Bridie Andrews (eds), *Western Medicine as Contested Knowledge*. Manchester University Press, 1997: 172–90.
12 James Clifford and George E. Marcus (eds), *Writing Culture: The Poetics and Politics of Ethnography*. Berkeley: University of California Press, 1986.
13 Edward W. Said, *Orientalism*. Harmondsworth: Penguin Books, 1985.
14 James Clifford. In *Writing Culture*, p. 12.
15 Ibid., p. 22.
16 To use examples from outside India, Peter Warwick and Bill Nasson focus on the

participation of black Africans, while Andrew Porter and others on British colonial servants. See Peter Warwick, *Black People and the South African War, 1899–1902*. Cambridge: Cambridge University Press, 1983; Bill Nasson, *Uyadela we' osulapho: Black Participation in the Anglo-Boer War*. Randburg: Ravan, 1999; A. N. Porter, *The Origins of the South African War: Joseph Chamberlain and the Diplomacy of Imperialism 1895–1899*. Manchester: Manchester University Press, 1980.

17 See for example, R. C. Richardson (compiler), *The Study of History: A Bibliographical Guide*. Manchester: Manchester University Press, 1988.

18 J. Hannam, A. Hughes, and P. Stafford (compilers), *British Women's History: A Bibliographical Guide*. Manchester: Manchester University Press, 1996.

19 Judith Walzer Leavitt, "'A Worrying Profession': The Domestic Environment of Medical Practice in Mid-19th-Century America." *Bulletin of the History of Medicine* (69 1995): 1–29.

20 A necessarily selective list might include (in chronological order): Norman G. Owen (ed.), *Death and Disease in South East Asia: Explorations in Social, Medical and Demographic History*. Singapore: Oxford University Press, 1987; David Arnold (ed.), *Imperial Medicine and Indigenous Societies*. Manchester University Press, 1988; Roy MacLeod and Milton Lewis (eds), *Disease, Medicine, and Empire. Perspectives on Western Medicine and the Experience of European Expansion*. London: Routledge, 1988; Megan Vaughan. *Curing Their Ills. Colonial Power and African Illness*. Cambridge: Polity Press, 1991; Poonam Bala, *Imperialism and Medicine in Bengal: A Sociohistorical Perspective*. New Delhi: Sage, 1991; Maryinez Lyons. *The Colonial Disease. A Social History of Sleeping Sickness in Northern Zaire, 1900–1940*. Cambridge: Cambridge University Press, 1992; Terence Ranger and Paul Slack (eds), *Epidemics and Ideas. Essays on the Historical Perception of Pestilence*. Cambridge: Cambridge University Press, 1992; Shirley Lindenbaum and Margaret Lock (eds), *Knowledge, Power and Practice: The Anthropology of Medicine and Everyday Life*. Berkeley: University of California Press, 1993; David Arnold, *Colonizing the Body. State Medicine and Epidemic Disease in Nineteenth-Century India*. Berkeley: University of California Press, 1993; Mark Harrison, *Public Health in British India: Anglo-Indian Preventive Medicine, 1859–1914*. Cambridge: Cambridge University Press, 1994; Marcos Cueto (ed.), *Missionaries of Science: The Rockefeller Foundation and Latin America*. Bloomington: Indiana University Press, 1994; Lenore Manderson, *Sickness and the State: Health and Illness in Colonial Malaya, 1870–1940*. Cambridge: Cambridge University Press, 1996; Andrew R. Cunningham and Bridie J. Andrews (eds), *Western Medicine as Contested Knowledge*. Manchester: Manchester University Press, 1997; Jonathan H. Sadowsky, *Imperial Bedlam: Institutions of Madness in Colonial Southwest Nigeria*. Berkeley: University of California Press, 1999.

21 Examples of works that observe medical pluralism include several of the contributions to Arthur Kleinman, Peter Kunstadter, E. Russell Alexander and James L. Cale (eds), *Medicine in Chinese Cultures: Comparative Studies of Health Care in Chinese and Other Societies*. Bethesda; National Institutes of Health, 1975; Charles Leslie and Allan Young (eds), *Paths to Asian Medical Knowledge*. Berkeley: University of California Press, 1990; Steven Feierman and John M. Janzen (eds), *The Social Basis of Health and Healing in Africa*. Berkeley: University of California Press, 1992.

22 Stuart Hall, "Who Needs 'Identity'?" In Stuart Hall and Paul du Gay (eds), *Questions of Cultural Identity*, London: Sage, 1996: 1–17.

23 On the history of state medical provision and public health, see George Rosen, *A History of Public Health. Expanded edition, with an Introduction by Elizabeth*

Fee. Baltimore: Johns Hopkins University Press, [1958] 1993; Barbara Rosenkrantz, *Public Health and the State: Changing Views in Massachusetts, 1842–1936*. Cambridge: Harvard University Press, 1972; Dorothy Porter (ed.), *The History of Public Health and the Modern State*. Wellcome Institute Series in the History of Medicine. Amsterdam: Rodopi, 1994.

24 JoAnn McGregor and Terence Ranger. "Displacement and Disease: Epidemics and Ideas About Malaria in Matabeleland, Zimbabwe, 1945–1996." *Past and Present* (167 1999): 203–37.

2 "The ignorance of women is the house of illness"
Gender, nationalism, and health reform in colonial north India

Maneesha Lal

> Nowadays one finds very few people who, whether educated or not, have a desire to learn about [the subject of childcare] and it is for this reason that the future builders of the nation die in such great numbers only a few days after their birth. . . . We should obtain [instruction in childcare] from the Western world. . . . By not continuing to shoulder their responsibilities in a complete manner [after their child is born, parents] become partners in a great sin which could be called a "National crime."
>
> Doctor Shrikant Tripathi[1]

> Nowadays we have fallen so in love with English knowledge that we disdain our excellent national customs that are thus day by day further deteriorating from neglect.
>
> Rameshwari Nehru[2]

By the early twentieth century, medical knowledge originating in the "West" had been circulating in India for several hundred years. "Western" medicine – or its various historical antecedents – arrived in India as part of more general historical processes of political expansion, trade, labor migration, cultural diffusion, and the extension of major religious traditions, and in this sense was no different from other medical and healing traditions which have spread via such means throughout history. Indians engaged with these Western medical traditions in numerous ways. Unani (*yånànā*) medical texts, describing the Graeco–Arabic system of medicine that was brought with Islam into India during the medieval period, were occasionally written in Sanskrit by scholars. Some Indians came into contact with Portuguese medical ideas and therapies in the 1500s. Ayurveda, a classical system of medicine that appears to have originated in Buddhist monasteries in India before being absorbed into the Hindu tradition, began reflecting disease descriptions common to Western medicine from the eighteenth century onwards. And from the very early days of the English East India Company's presence in India, certain Indians encountered Western medicine by working as assistants and orderlies in its hospitals.[3]

As the British were bringing ever larger portions of the Indian subcontinent under their military and political control during the eighteenth and nineteenth centuries, Western medicine began to play an increasingly central role in shaping the self-identity of British as well as other European societies. Heralded as an emblem of benevolence and civilization, medicine served a powerful function in legitimizing the colonizing process and facilitating imperial dominance over indigenous populations in cultural and social as well as scientific domains. As a knowledge system which increasingly claimed unique access to truth about the body, health, and disease, Western medicine operated as a potent discursive and instrumental means by which Indian and other colonized populations were represented and defined – most often, of course, in negative terms.[4] Colonial doctors typically depicted "natives" as dirty, ignorant, and superstitious, thereby authorizing assumptions of racial and cultural superiority. Asian and African healing specialists – and the forms of medicine they practiced – began to be routinely denounced, viewed as barbaric and unscientific, while Western medical practice was presumed to rest on an enlightened and rational basis. Western medicine thus helped to constitute fundamental aspects of European identity in the age of empire.[5]

Turning to the specific case of India, a growing body of scholarship has pointed to the influential role of Western medical discourse and practice in underwriting ideologies of British superiority during the "high noon" period of colonial rule. We also have evidence of interactions between such groups as Indian students and British missionary physicians; Ayurvedic practitioners and Indian Medical Service officers; Indian women plague sufferers and British male public health authorities. Yet scholars have been cautious about claiming that Western medicine had significant and widespread impact on the majority of the Indian population, or that it fundamentally shaped Indian notions of identity. Debate concerning the reasons for this presumed limited impact has tended to stress either British enclavism and frugality or Indian ignorance and resistance.[6]

Indeed the nature and extent of Western medicine's impact on the self-identities, perceptions, and practices of the Indian population still remain largely a matter of speculation, for earlier periods as well as for the nineteenth and twentieth centuries. Careful exploration is required of an array of sources representing a variety of perspectives – including those of groups marginalized by structures of dominance within Indian society and differentiated by gender, region, language, caste, class, and religion, among other factors, in order to give any more general claims substantial foundation.[7]

In this chapter, I examine the engagement of Indian women and men with the ideological underpinnings and therapeutic implications of Western medicine by focusing on articles on the topics of health, hygiene, and medicine that were published in the Hindi women's magazine *Stri Darpan* (*Strā Darpaō*).[8] Founded in 1909 by Rameshwari Nehru, *Stri Darpan*, or "The Mirror of Women," became one of the leading Hindi women's journals of the early twentieth century. Aimed at the growing numbers of middle and upper-class women who were becoming literate in the new Hindi prose language, *Stri Darpan* addressed important social and political issues of the day, including women's education, legal reform, suffrage, and Indian independence. Serious about its educational mission and proud of its unique feminist and nationalist perspective, *Stri Darpan* reflected and participated in debates concerning cultural identities in north India at a time when those identities were undergoing significant reformulation and change. That the magazine devoted considerable attention to the subjects of health and medicine on its pages provokes several questions regarding the relationships between medicine and identity in this particular north Indian context: What was the nature of the medical models being promoted in *Stri Darpan*, and what role did they play in articulating new cultural identities? Did the imperatives and desires of nationalism shape Indian understandings of medical traditions and concerns about the health of Indian women? How were Indian women positioned in these new discourses of hygiene and health – as patients, as healers, as citizen-mothers? And to what extent were medical conceptions tied to other processes of identity formation – such as those involving language, class, caste, and religion – that were linked to Indian nationalism and characterized colonial north India in the early decades of the twentieth century?

I examine these questions within multiple contexts: the rise of the early twentieth-century Indian women's organizations; the development of the Hindi prose language; the spread of new forms of vernacular print production addressed to female audiences; and the growth of movements to revitalize Ayurveda. My analysis presumes the view advanced in recent scholarship that cultural identities – and indeed national identities – are imagined, engineered, and invented, that far from transcending time or place they are contingent historical products and the result of ideological and cultural work.[9] Exploring the specific historical and social structural contexts that gave rise to new linked identities in early twentieth-century north India enables us to see *Stri Darpan* – and the medical conceptions it promoted – as intimately tied to the broader social historical processes of middle-class formation, the re-articulation of patriarchies, and the consolidation of nationalism.

Rameshwari Nehru and *Stri Darpan*

Stri Darpan was founded by Rameshwari Nehru in Allahabad, the seat of the Nehru family dynasty, a political center of the twentieth-century nationalist movement, and the most important city for women's education in Hindi speaking regions.[10] Rameshwari had arrived in the city in 1902, upon her marriage at the age of sixteen to the Oxford-educated Brijlal Nehru, the youngest son of Jawaharlal Nehru's eldest paternal uncle. Rameshwari hailed from an aristocratic family descended from Kashmiri Brahmins who had long settled in Lahore; her father, Raja Narendranath, served as a high-ranking government officer and later became Member of the Legislative Assembly in Punjab as well as President of the All-India Hindu Mahasabha (Hindu Great Association). Raja Narendranath was a proud man who admired elements of British civilization and rule while maintaining faith in many Indian traditions and moral values. When Rameshwari reached the age of twelve, for example, her father insisted that she observe *purdah* (*pardà*, veiling and seclusion).[11] Yet at a time when the education of girls was rare, Rameshwari, along with her four sisters, received a good education at home from the governess appointed to her brother. While still in Lahore, she met Muhammadi Begam, who had founded a women's association devoted to social reform and edited the weekly Urdu newspaper for women *Tahzib un-Niswan* (The Women's Reformer).[12]

When Rameshwari arrived in Allahabad as the newest member of the Anglicized Nehru extended family, she was well-educated and forward-looking for her time. She knew Hindi and Urdu well, spoke and read very widely in English, and also commanded some Persian and Sanskrit. The patriotic and feminist leanings Rameshwari had developed earlier from reading magazines, newspapers, and biographies gained strength and conviction in the welcoming soil of Anand Bhavan (Abode of Happiness), the grand home built by Motilal Nehru, Jawaharlal Nehru's father and the family patriarch. Purdah was not observed at Anand Bhavan, and women in the Nehru family were apparently treated according to new ideals of modernity and equality. In 1906, Rameshwari, barely twenty, posted a letter to Jawaharlal Nehru, then at Harrow School in England. In it she implored him to "Return soon to India – your motherland is waiting for you so that you liberate her and alleviate her suffering."[13]

Rameshwari Nehru became a central figure in the women's movement and nationalist movement in north India. With the assistance of her sister-in-law Uma Nehru and other women of the Nehru extended family, Rameshwari continued as editor of *Stri Darpan* for over a decade after its inauguration.[14] She also founded the Prayag Mahila Samiti (Allahabad Women's Association) in 1909, organized meetings to raise women's consciousness about such issues as anti-Indian discrimination in South Africa, and established a forum where young girls could gain skills in debate and discussion. Later, she was the only woman invited to serve on the Age of Consent Committee, which was set up by the British government in 1927 to examine pending social legislation on issues of child marriage and the age of consent. Rameshwari gained prominence for her work with the committee and with nationalist women's organizations, particularly the Women's India Association. She soon became closely linked to Mahatma Gandhi, especially after becoming involved at his request in the movement for the uplift of untouchables. Rameshwari served for numerous Indian women as their "ideal of Indian womanhood" – humble, lovable, and selfless, yet energetically devoted to a productive, public life based on Gandhian ideals.[15]

In comparison with Bengal, Maharashtra, and Madras, the Hindi region in north India was less active in campaigning and organizing around issues concerning women; only in the twentieth century did the women's movement make any significant impact in Hindi-speaking provinces.[16] *Stri Darpan* was critical to this effort, surpassing the many other early twentieth century women's magazines in the seriousness and depth with which it examined women's issues. Vir Bharat Talwar has argued that while there were at least five Hindi women's journals of differing perspectives published at the time, *Stri Darpan* "became the most important instrument in the women's movement in the Hindi provinces."[17] Vijaya Lakshmi Pandit, Jawaharlal Nehru's sister and herself a prominent political figure, described *Stri Darpan* in her memoirs as:

> The equal in content of any modern woman's magazine published in America or the United Kingdom – probably better, since it dealt with subjects important to the Indian woman such as the need for better education, inheritance, abolition of child marriage, divorce, remarriage of widows, and the right to vote.[18]

Editorials and articles in *Stri Darpan* carried such titles as "Why Doesn't India's Progress Occur?" "The Socialist Tradition," "Child Marriage and Its Harmful Social Effects," "Women and the Vote," "Christianity and Ancient India," "Women and Self-Rule," "The Diet of English Soldiers," and "Women and Social Liberty." Along with numerous articles concerning topics of health and hygiene, such titles reflect the journal's goal of providing serious, pedagogical fare to its women readers and contributing to their political awakening in both public and private spheres. *Stri Darpan*'s circulation appears to have remained relatively small, never more than 1,000 copies according to a recent estimate.[19] While the full extent of the journal's impact remains unclear, there is considerable evidence that Indian newspapers and journals circulated much more widely – by, for example, being passed around to friends and relations or being read aloud in public – than their official figures would suggest.[20] Given the limited numbers of literate women in India at the time, *Stri Darpan*'s content provides a valuable index of what its editors and authors assumed were important issues for north Indian women. Advertising itself in 1919 as "the only journal which teaches women rights along with their dharma (*duty*) because husbands, brothers and fathers cannot promote the welfare of the country while treating women like animals," *Stri Darpan* communicated a clear feminist – and nationalist – consciousness.[21] Yet it represented and accommodated a range of distinctive viewpoints. The journal contained, for example, a number of scathing articles by Uma Nehru, articulating a version of equal-rights feminism, rejecting mainstream nationalist symbols of femininity based on Hindu scriptural models such as Sita, Sati, and Savitri, and adopting a European-based outlook. Editor Rameshwari Nehru's views, however, were more in line with those of Mahatma Gandhi. Nehru and Gandhi promoted a reformed ideal for women seen to be more realistically suited to Indian conditions and goals.[22]

The contexts of the rise of women's journalism and women's organizations, as well as the development of Hindi as a prose language, are crucial for understanding the role and significance of *Stri Darpan* in early twentieth-century north India. By the late nineteenth and early twentieth centuries, Indian women across the country had begun forming independent organizations, as part of what some scholars have labeled "a growing and active feminist movement."[23] These groups differed from the nineteenth-century social reform movements that had been led by men for "women's uplift" and had focused on promotion of widow remarriage, raising the age of consent, and abolition of *satā* (the burning of a Hindu widow on the funeral pyre of her husband). These new women's groups, by contrast, set up institutions to educate widows and destitute women, engage in social reform, and educate and edify their members.[24] Initially city or regionally based, such as the Prayag Mahila Samiti established by Rameshwari Nehru in 1909, by the late 1920s several organizations claimed to be active on an all-India level. In their antagonism to the colonial state and their analysis of its inadequacies, the middle and upper-class, upper-caste Indian women who participated in such national associations reconceptualized their place in the new imagined nation. Yet from their privileged social location they were often unable to identify with the oppressions and constraints that less privileged women faced. Indeed, in many cases, these women positioned themselves for the tasks of the new national woman by distinguishing themselves from lower class and caste Hindu women, Muslim, and Western women. And they remained for the most part circumscribed by the nationalist movement, which articulated a reformist modernizing agenda – for example by agreeing in 1919 to women's suffrage – but also constrained women's emancipation within a modified patriarchy.[25]

A number of scholars have argued that "the women's question," which had figured prominently in the nineteenth-century movements of social reform in India, was superseded in the latter decades of the century by the new – and more narrowly political – concerns of nationalism.[26] This argument does not take into account the proliferation of new forms of writing that served as important arenas for continued debate concerning women's role and position in society. By the latter half of the nineteenth century, privileged women in many parts of India began writing stories and autobiographies in significantly greater numbers, and publishing journals and magazines for themselves.[27] Between the 1880s and 1920s, Susie Tharu and K. Lalita argue, "the women's question" of the nineteenth century did not disappear but was "enthusiastically carried forward, expanded, and transformed by women. All over the country women had hardly begun to read and write before they were editing and publishing in journals that had surprisingly long runs."[28] Hundreds of women began contributing articles, poems, and stories in languages such as Bengali, English, Telugu, Kannada,

Gujarati, Urdu, and Hindi, to journals whose readership was predominantly female. The early twentieth century clearly marked an unprecedented period in women's journalism, characterized by a more radical and critical outlook compared to the reformist phase of the nineteenth century.[29] Representing the convergence of several factors, including the diffusion of women's education, the spread of certain institutions and modes of print capitalism, and the development of the prose vernacular languages, these journals form rich sources for approaching questions concerning identity formation. As Rosalind O'Hanlon has remarked,

> Historians have long appreciated the extent to which later nineteenth century vernacular literatures were important vehicles for a range of religious and regional political identities. It is only more recently that we have begun to discover their significance in the construction of gender identities.[30]

I would argue, moreover, that these vernacular literatures were integral to the shaping of medical – and national – identities as well.

The development of the Hindi prose language, in which the journal *Stri Darpan* was written, was the result of a complex set of changes in education, administration, communication, and political mobilization set in motion by both Britons and Indians over the course of the nineteenth and early twentieth centuries. A marked plurality of languages and dialects had characterized north Indian society in earlier decades. Persian had been the language of the Mughal court, and the popular north Indian language was Hindustani, with Urdu its Persianized, refined form written in the Persian script.[31] The British, as part of their efforts to expand their growing power on the subcontinent, had begun compiling dictionaries and grammars of Indian languages, including Hindustani, in the late eighteenth century. In the 1830s, the colonial administration replaced Persian with Urdu as the official court language and installed English as the language of public instruction. Yet Hindi, virtually identical to Urdu in grammar and phonology though written in Devanagari (*Devanàgarā*), the script used most frequently for Sanskrit, began receiving support shortly thereafter from the colonial army and missionaries, as well as from Indian princes, commercial communities, and Hindu religious reformers. The spread of printing technology in the region in the 1830s and 1840s encouraged the standardization of Hindi, and later decades witnessed its growth and evolution as it adapted new Western prose genres such as essays, novels, and short stories.[32] Among these works were a number of books on the topics of medicine, surgery, and hygiene, ranging from classical Ayurvedic texts and medical lexicons to compilations of Indian plants and drugs and books dealing specifically with diseases of women.[33]

By the last decades of the century, Hindi became a focus of controversies over linguistic, regional, and religious identities in north India. Upper-caste, middle-class Hindi literati sought to replace Urdu and English with Hindi in the administration and schools, to challenge the upholders of Urdu as well as the advantaged English-educated Bengali élites who had settled in the region. Hindi promoters – merchants, teachers, scholars, lawyers, and publicists, among others – were also active in furthering a Hindu-based sense of community in opposition to Muslims and Christians, and traced their roots back to what they perceived as their authentic Aryan origins. Through institutions such as the Nagari Pracharini Sabha (Society for the Printing of Nagari), founded in Banaras in 1893, and the Hindi Sahitya Sammelan (Society for Hindi Literature), founded in 1910 in Allahabad, Hindi intellectuals engaged in constructing a literary canon, promoting a *suddh* (pure) version of the Hindi language, and publishing suitable Hindi books, including those on medicine and science. Supporters of Hindi advanced its claims as a potential national language, as capable of forging new bonds of sentiment that would shed the domination of English and represent a distinctively Indian essence. Meanwhile, publications in Hindi proliferated throughout the towns of northern India.

In the realm of magazine publishing, *Sarasvati (Sarasvatā)* became the best known and most popular and influential of the Hindi magazines established during the early twentieth century. Founded in 1900 in Allahabad, it flourished under the editorship of Mahavirprasad Dvivedi from 1903–20. Through his tireless efforts selecting and editing submissions he deemed suitable for improving the character of his Hindi readers, Dvivedi played a major role in establishing a standard form of Hindi prose. The success of *Sarasvati*, whose subject matter emphasized science and history as well as literature, encouraged other literary activity, and journals particularly took on vital educative functions as arenas for political debate and literary expression. Many of them, like *Stri Darpan*, were designed to cater to the needs of newly literate middle and upper-class women, who in the Hindi provinces were slowly following their Bengali counterparts into the colonial public sphere.[34] In 1918, when a Hindi Literature Conference was organized in the city of Indore, 700 women took part in a session chaired by Mahatma Gandhi to discuss literature in Hindi and topics such as "Literature suitable for women in the Hindi language."[35]

The new form of written Hindi that was being promoted, however, had been stripped of its Urdu and Perso-Arabic heritage and vocabulary (now deemed foreign) and injected with Sanskrit loan-words and more complex syntax; it was also disassociated from the other spoken varieties of the region. Thus, while Hindi supporters claimed a more popular mass-based appeal for the language, arguing that it was far better than English as the vehicle for mass education and the spread of both modern ideas and Indian cultural identity, the new *suddh* Hindi served to discriminate against lower castes and Muslims and became the language of another élite, accessible to a relatively limited section of north Indian society. Hindi was thus similar to other national languages, such as Italian or French, which were also the result of controversy, subjected to processes of selection, demarcation, and purification, and initially confined to small portions of their populations.[36]

Identifying nationalist medical traditions

Stri Darpan thus reflected and participated in the complex processes of identity formation that characterized northern India in the early twentieth century. Medical and hygienic ideas played an important role in the struggle over and elaboration of these new identities, both within the pages of *Stri Darpan* and in various other forums. With its numerous articles containing advice on health maintenance, information about specific diseases or disorders, and counsel on childbirth and childcare, *Stri Darpan* reflected the desire of an emerging regional middle-class, constituted by recently forged bonds of linguistic kinship, to reconstruct strong bodily identities that could withstand the demands of nation building and self-rule in modern times. Stung by British reprehension of Indian medical and sanitary practices and concerned about health conditions in their country, *Stri Darpan* authors sought to fashion for themselves and their readers a new corporeal consciousness geared to the requirements of the imagined Indian nation, a nation in which certain class, caste, gender, and religious hierarchies were being reinscribed *and* remade. The elements for constructing this new consciousness were selected and adapted from existing healing traditions – themselves arrayed along hierarchies of power and degrees of accessibility – which were scrutinized and evaluated for this nation-building task.

Stri Darpan accommodated two distinct medical idioms, one derived from Ayurvedic knowledge traditions and the other relying on Western medical frameworks of understanding. These models were clearly reflected in authors' choice of medical topics, notions about health, conceptions of the body, and ideas of disease causation. Yet despite important differences between the two models of healing, all authors writing on health issues in *Stri Darpan* emphasized the important role of Indian women in the national body project, as protectors, once appropriately educated, of the health of their families and thereby the health of the nation.

Consistent with Indian nationalism's quest for cultural regeneration in a perceived ancient Hindu Golden Age, several of the articles in *Stri Darpan* sought to actively identify, revitalize, and disseminate for their female readers a nationalist "tradition" of medicine in the form of Ayurveda. Since authors adapted their presentations of Ayurvedic precepts for the *Stri Darpan* audience, their articles rarely delved into the detailed complexities of Ayurvedic thought. Rather, they configured a more popular version of hygienic principles and accessible advice meant for their increasingly educated, semi-literate, middle-class audience. The authorities invoked to support this re-awakening medical culture included Ayurvedic texts such as the *Caraka Samhita* and *Susruta Samhita*, other unnamed "ancient texts," and ancestors and old rituals and customs. Authors bemoaned the fact that contemporary youth and educated authorities regarded their ancient knowledge as useless and thus were sacrificing themselves to Western civilization.[37] As Rameshwari Nehru put it, in a notice about a woman who had gained enormous strength from her practice of *pràōàyàm* (yogic breath exercises), "Nowadays we have fallen so in love with English knowledge that we disdain our excellent national customs that are thus day by day further deteriorating from neglect."[38]

The body, in this Ayurvedic model, was constructed out of three humors – *vàt* (wind), *pittà* (bile), and *kaph* (phlegm) – which could each become agitated or displaced and provoke ill health.[39] Health thus depended on the constant equilibrium of these humors, and was maintained by proper diet and regimen. Food was categorized according to humoral type and was to be taken according to the ideal of appropriateness, to time and place, to season, to region and nation, and to the particular constitution and temperament of individual bodies.[40] Months and seasons were seen as having characteristic humoral influences, necessitating the avoidance of particular foods, emotions, and behaviors in order to counteract potential adverse effects.[41] For example, Prem Dulari argued that during the months of *Asoj* and *Kàrttik*, when *pittà* asserted its power, it was important to abstain from yogurt, pungent oil, and salty foodstuffs and to refrain from eating too much, getting angry, or staying too long in the sun. Dulari also invoked the Ayurvedic tenet that certain foods are incompatible and unhealthy in combination, warning, for example, against mixing honey together with *ghā* (clarified butter).[42]

The centrality of physiological processes of digestion in the Ayurvedic conception of the body was also reflected in *Stri Darpan* articles. Many authors presented as axiomatic the Ayurvedic-derived idea that digestion, understood as *agni* (fire), sustains life, and that *mal* (waste matter) if improperly eliminated could spread via the blood as poison throughout the body.[43] Everyday analogies were often used to simplify and make accessible more complex concepts. For example, B. K. Mitra claimed that the body could be understood as a *càlhà*, or open stove, which in order to function properly had to have its ashes (the body's waste products) regularly removed.[44] Digestive problems could result from a variety of causes, including delayed mealtimes, improper diet, insufficient exercise, worry or anger, or excessive mental stimulation. With entire articles devoted to indigestion, constipation, overeating, and discussion of food preparation and cooking, *Stri Darpan* was resonant with the concerns of Hindu popular culture – itself influenced by widespread Ayurvedic precepts – of the need to micromanage the complex processes of bodily intake, absorption, and elimination.[45] The Ayurvedic body, envisioned as a complex hydraulic system constantly in flux due to a combination of changing emotional states, necessary bodily functions, climatic and seasonal conditions, and moral and behavioral choices, required a regimen devoted to managing possible adverse influences and thereby ensuring a stable equilibrium.

Moral and sacred duty could coincide with proper bodily practice. The body and mind were understood as an integrated whole with each necessarily influencing the other. For example, Shri Jagannath Shukla asserted that singing hymns in the early morning was beneficial not only because one increased one's musical knowledge and remembered the Lord's name, but also because music made the *dil* (heart/spirit) happy and thus calmed the nerves of the stomach. Rising at dawn, defecating, washing the mouth and face, bathing, singing hymns, practicing breath control, performing sacred rituals – all were religious prescriptions necessarily aligned with the elements of healthful living. Fasts performed on such occasions as *ekādaśī, śivrātri,* and other holy days, were said to have originated partly from the need that ancestors had recognized, to restore bodily balance after suffering bouts of indigestion, constipation or other disorders. As Shukla rhetorically asked, "Does this mean there is a connecting link between the *dharmaśāstras* [Hindu treatises on sacred duty/'law'], and the *ārogyaśāstras* [treatises on health]? Necessarily there is."[46]

To ensure a proper appreciation of Ayurveda's virtues and of India's heritage, it was vital, *Stri Darpan* authors insisted, that this ancient medical tradition be better understood and promoted. The trope of loss, of earlier Ayurvedic knowledge being supplanted by *óàkñarā* medicine (the term used to refer to Western medicine) or only continuing to exist in dry ritualistic form, underscored the need for revitalizing efforts.[47] Rameshwari Nehru consistently adopted a nationalist perspective that argued for patronage of Ayurveda and further exploration of its likely benefits. In a review of the first book published on the subject of childbirth and maternity in Hindi, Nehru noted approvingly that the author quoted important extracts from Ayurveda's classical texts and compared Ayurvedic theories with *óàkñarā* medicine to demonstrate that the craft of childbirth was in an advanced state in ancient India. Yet Nehru complained that the book did not mention the names of any Ayurvedic germ-killing medicines and listed only *óàkñarā* drugs. She found it difficult to believe that Ayurveda did not contain such drugs, and argued that more research was needed on this topic.[48]

In implicit, if not explicitly acknowledged, tension with the Ayurvedic model, a Western medical model occupied a prominent role in *Stri Darpan* as well. Authors writing in this mode often claimed the title "Doctor" and indicated qualifications from Indian medical schools by appending the initials of L.M.P. (Licensed Medical Practitioner) or L.M.S. (Licentiate in Medicine and Surgery) to their names. Their articles dwelt primarily on issues of infant and maternal mortality, midwifery training, and proper methods of childbirth and childcare. Making hierarchical comparisons with other countries regarding India's rates of infant and maternal mortality, authors such as Shrikant Tripathi argued forcefully that knowledge of childcare and hygiene should be obtained from the Western world. Otherwise, parents would become partners in a great sin which could be called a "National crime."[49] The Oxford graduate Shriyut Mukandilal warned that in the current age of the "struggle for existence," if India's little boys and girls were not raised to become healthy, robust, and independent, as were children in England and other foreign lands, the Indian community would become extinct like the old Egyptians and Romans or like the Red Indians of America.[50] Westernizing authors blamed illiteracy, fatalistic attitudes, faulty medical treatment, ignorance of proper childcare methods, lack of skilled midwives, and societal and parental – especially maternal – negligence for the overwhelming pervasiveness of infant disease and death.[51]

Indigenous customs and traditions came under particular attack. Although Doctor Shrikant Tripathi acknowledged that poverty often increased vulnerability to disease and death, he complained that in India wealth did not ensure greater protection from such tragedies. Tripathi argued that wealthy Indian parents seemed to think overfeeding their children was a sign of affection and prestige. "You will not be able to see this in any English home," he declared, adding ironically, "Perhaps English people love children less! Love's aim is not to kill [children] by overfeeding them."[52] Internalizing a dominant element of the colonial critique, Tripathi asserted,

> A country's social customs and traditions have an effect on its inhabitants. In some places [those social customs] raise the mental strength of their people; in others they make their people energetic and courageous. But in this country the misfortune is that [our customs and traditions] are not satisfied only in making our unfortunate stock cowardly and contemptible, but moreover act as a very deadly poison on tiny babies.[53]

Tripathi identified the joint family as a distinctively Indian institution that served as the locus of social hierarchies that often undermined the health of its members. Normative patterns of deference and humility in the presence of elders and a complexly calibrated economy of relations considered necessary to maintain the joint family's smooth operation militated against husbands and wives singling out each other or their own children for special attention or care. As Tripathi argued, the regrettable result of this was that a man would be severely ostracized if he looked after the care and nourishment of his wife and children and made arrangements for their medical treatment if sick. Not only would he be seen to be acting contrary to proper methods of obtaining merit and status, but his behavior would also be considered a sign of *Ghor Kaliyug*, the final and most debased of the four eras posited in classical Hinduism.[54] Young daughters-in-law were also said to be subject to intense social pressure, being discouraged by fear or shame from consulting their mothers-in-law for advice regarding their newly-born children.[55]

If the Ayurvedic model emphasized physiological processes, the *ḋākñarā* idiom stressed anatomy, as well as certain conceptual, institutional, and therapeutic elements consistent with a Western medical model. The names of specific organs were translated phonetically into the Devanagari script from English, with occasional terms and phrases written in English itself. Organs were introduced and explained in terms of their function and location, indicating that authors were self-consciously presenting anatomical terminology they presumed unfamiliar to their audience.[56] The gaseous composition of air and the properties of oxygen, nitrogen, and carbonic acid gas were described in plain and simple terms in an article emphasizing the importance of clean air, clean water, and clean food for maintaining health.[57] The occasional mention of "germ-killing" medicines indicated at least superficial familiarity with germ theory, and germs of cholera and typhoid were acknowledged to exist even in the sacred river Ganges.[58] Young women and widows interested in midwifery were advised to obtain formal institutional education in medical colleges and schools following the *óākñarā* model, and to secure certificates from those schools and municipalities or hospitals to attest to the completion of their training. They were instructed to submit to the authority of qualified doctors. Prospective midwives were told they would need to learn how to use tools such as the thermometer, which was described as an instrument to see fever, and the catheter, described as an instrument to remove waste; again, the English terms for these instruments were transliterated into Devanagari script.[59] Therapeutic admonitions were concerned less with regulation of diet and digestion than with the use of "proper" medicines – that is, those supplied by practitioners of Western medicine.[60]

The implicitly, if not explicitly, dual model of medicine being promoted in *Stri Darpan* suggests that Western medicine circulated widely and influenced many Indians' understandings of their bodily strengths and capacities. It also points to the widespread impact of the Ayurvedic revitalization movements, which were at their height in the first decades of the twentieth century. Ayurvedic practitioners had from the early years of British rule adopted elements of Western medicine into their own thought and practice – a process we still know little about. Yet they suffered from a loss of political patronage as the colonial government became increasingly disdainful of Indian medicine as the nineteenth century progressed. From the 1880s and 1890s, practitioners of Ayurvedic medicine, inspired by Orientalist ideology which postulated a glorious ancient Indian civilization that had suffered decline, sought to revitalize their medical traditions by adopting institutional forms, ideas, and technology from the Western medical tradition. The first professional interest group of indigenous practitioners, the All-India Ayurvedic Congress, was established in 1907. Medical colleges as well as pharmaceutical companies were founded in different parts of the country. To publicize their efforts and provide curricula for the new colleges, Ayurvedic practitioners translated classical Sanskrit texts into English and vernacular languages, and began publishing textbooks and journals.[61]

By the second decade of the twentieth century, provincial governments in Bombay, Bengal, and Madras capitulated to recurrent campaigns by Indian Medical Service officers – by now increasingly Indian – and established Medical Registration Acts. These enabled only registered practitioners of

Western medicine to hold hospital or government posts and imposed fines on offenders. In 1921, as medicine was transferred to provincial governments under dyarchy as part of the Montagu–Chelmsford reforms, Ayurvedic practitioners relied on nationalist arguments to gain the support of some, if not all, of the newly appointed Indian ministers. With the backing of sympathetic Indian ministers and some members of the nationalist movement, revitalizers also lobbied government agencies to gain support for research and training in Ayurveda. These revitalization movements were marked by conflicts, however. Advocates of a "pure" Ayurveda wished to eliminate use of modern technologies and teach only from ancient and medieval texts, while those who argued for an integrated medical system were ready to incorporate elements of Western medicine and its technological armamentarium to improve Ayurvedic practice.[62] *Stri Darpan*'s eclectic and inclusive editorial policy suggested support for an integrated system, combining an appreciation of Ayurvedic medicine as well as a willingness to accept some elements of Western medicine.

"The ignorance of women is the house of illness"

Common to both the Ayurvedic and Western idioms as presented in *Stri Darpan* was the special role and responsibility accorded middle-class women. As Prem Dulari proclaimed: "A person's health is in the hands of women . . . *Striyoṁ kā ajñān bīmārī kā ghar hai* [The ignorance of women is the house of illness]." Women's carelessness, negligence, and ignorance – all were identified as primary causes of deaths, particularly those of children. In her article, which singled out poor diet as the cause of a majority of all deaths, Dulari ultimately blamed mothers' ignorance of proper nutrition as the cause of death in young children. In graphic language, she proclaimed that bad diets caused:

> New buds . . . [to] wither and die even before they have a chance to blossom. Thousands of mothers, who after great anticipation have welcomed a tiny child into their houses, are beset with grief, but those poor [women] do not realize that all this is the result only of their own ignorance.[63]

In an article originally published in *Modern Review* and translated into Hindi for *Stri Darpan*, Sundarimohan Das, M. B., rhapsodized that in India motherhood was always regarded as the highest function of female life and that most Indian women still wished to become mothers despite the recent influence of "pernicious" birth control propaganda from the West. Quoting from a Sanskrit text to illustrate how in Hinduism even God had been represented as "having taken birth as a human babe to taste a mother's love," Das nevertheless lamented that contemporary Indian mothers were unprepared for their exalted work. He approvingly introduced an extract of a speech given by Mrs William Lowell Putnam, who as president of the American Association for the Study and Prevention of Infant Mortality had, Das claimed, called for girls to be properly trained in the tasks of motherhood and homemaking. Das argued that only with such training would Indian women be able to save their babies from preventable diseases and death.[64]

Stri Darpan authors conceived of the lack of knowledge, or lack of concern or interest that they attributed to women (and occasionally also to men), in national terms, as characterizing and implicitly distinguishing *hamārā deś* or *rāṣṭra* (our country, nation) from others in the world community.[65] As Dipesh Chakrabarty has noted, "The civilising discourse that propelled . . . nationalist thought thus produced the figure of the 'uneducated housewife/mother' as one of its central problems."[66] Yet the possibility of "improvement," of "education," implied that India could take her place among the world's nations, secure in her characteristic distinctiveness yet striving simultaneously toward modernity. If properly educated, *Stri Darpan* authors assured Indian women, they could restore sick persons to health and save others from becoming ill. Such knowledgeable women could also prevent unscrupulous doctors from taking advantage of members of their communities.[67] *Stri Darpan* readers were encouraged to purchase and read books and advice literature on topics such as childbirth and maternity, and to be active agents in the maintenance of their own – and particularly others' – health. The editorial office served as a distribution center for self-help manuals the editor considered especially valuable, with special promotions arranged with authors.[68] Articles such as "Some Necessary Points Concerning Childcare" presented lists of simple exhortatory statements, urging readers not to cough or sneeze in front of infants, nor to promenade with babies in bad air or excessive sun, nor to expose them to flies and mosquitoes. Authors relied heavily on Hindi grammatical forms which indicated obligation and desirability – the equivalents of "ought" or "should" – in constructing their sentences. The ideal mother, according to this literature, was one who fed her child at the same time every day, had him vaccinated in his first year, breastfed him knowing it was the best nourishment, and never gave him any medicine without the advice of a doctor or *vaid* (Ayurvedic physician).[69] *Stri Darpan* thus promoted a guided, expert-led and assisted health reform.

Yet as Partha Chatterjee has pointed out, while the identity of the new woman fashioned by nationalist discourse was constructed in contrast to uneducated women of earlier generations as well as to lower-class women, the fear that Indian women would become too Westernized was also an all-pervasive one.[70] Such anxieties and fears were clearly reflected in *Stri Darpan*'s articles, in which the discourse of hygiene often incorporated disapproving assumptions about *sabhyatā*, or civilization. Authors claimed that the adoption of "civilized" habits – such as following a more sedentary lifestyle and a richer diet along with a corresponding reduction in individual labor – led to disease. In his article on constipation, for example, Shriyut B. K. Mitra cited civilization itself as the root cause of this disorder. Substituting a vegetable diet with a diet rich in meats, sweets, and fats, as well as replacing bodily labor with mental labor meant for Mitra that the power of intestines to expel feces – a major concern within the Ayurvedic worldview – had slackened.[71] In his article on women and tuberculosis in India, Shri Mukutvihari Lal Dar expressed shame and concern about the excessively high incidence of tuberculosis morbidity and mortality among Indian's women. Yet Dar also reflected widespread anxieties about the effects of modern Western civilization on the purity, devotion, and self-sacrifice of women whose primary responsibility was still to serve family and nation. Dar reproached "fashionable ladies" for neglecting their traditional home duties, reading sentimental novels, succumbing to nervous excitement, and becoming slaves of fashion, and linked these to a decreased bodily resistance to tuberculosis. To combat tuberculosis, Dar encouraged women's household labor:

> Our well-born ladies . . . should definitely work, because the means of getting rid of tuberculosis is bodily labor. Showing enthusiasm for housework, sweeping our rooms and keeping them clean, washing our clothes and mending them, pounding paddy in our house with a *dheṁkī*, grinding flour with light flourmills, pulling water from a well and preparing food for our husbands, dear children and mother and father – from doing all this and other household work with our own hands, our lungs will enlarge and we will remain in good health. From this, work will be done properly and lower expenditure will result – and, the most important thing is this – that the people in the household will get wholesome, pure, and good food, due to which there will be respite from fears of indigestion or constipation. I do not stop our young girls from blameless amusements of the heart/mind, but loving service always bestows happiness, and by serving her family without feelings of resentment but full of love, every woman makes herself into a true daughter of the almighty supreme being.[72]

Other authors addressed fears of excessive Westernization by attempting to re-acquaint Indian women with their ostensible heritage. For example, Doctor Mahendralal Garg stated that the Matsya Purana, one of a group of ancient Hindu sacred texts, contained advice truly beneficial for women about how to obtain a good son. Included in Garg's select list of instructions were the following pithy admonitions: a woman [desiring a good son] should not exercise, keep her hair untied, wear soaked clothing, utter inauspicious remarks, or quarrel with her husband or with other men.[73] The flexible discourse of hygiene and disease could easily meld desired gender, class, and national identities into its prescriptive agenda.

Taken in sum, the articles in *Stri Darpan* suggest that the practice of health care, at least among some members of the urban élite, was very gradually and unevenly making the transition from embodied domestic knowledge, residing with older women of individual households and certain decentralized healing specialists, to a more codified, formalized body of knowledge to be dispensed by individual (primarily male) doctors and other self-proclaimed authorities. Authors often invoked the widespread lack of knowledge regarding preparation of medicines and medical treatment and care, presenting it as a particularly contemporary dilemma. As B. K. Mitra remarked in his article on *ajārō* (indigestion), "in previous times, old women would prepare medicines for common diseases by themselves but with the advent of *òàkñarā* medicine that practice has nearly become extinct."[74] A doctor, Prasadilal Jha, L.M.S., complained that the reason trained midwives were now necessary was because while "old ladies of our houses" used to know something or other about childbirth and its management, now the young women, old ladies of the towns, and even many existing midwives, "knew nothing." The result of this loss of expertise, Jha asserted, was that after giving birth women's lives were often ruined by disease, or they and their children died even in the lying-in chamber.[75] The practical basis and moral justification for such instruction as *Stri Darpan* authors advocated was predicated on the assumption of their female readers' ignorance – and hence need. Although *Stri Darpan*'s readers were granted an important role in this reformist effort, as individual wives and mothers with primary responsibility for their families' health and thus the health of the nation, they were to be led and advised in this project by self-styled experts. As certain domains of medicine moved very gradually into the hands of a trained élite and centralized institutions – of both the Ayurvedic and Western medical varieties – some women likely began to lose a measure of the autonomy and authority they had earlier possessed in this arena.[76]

In keeping with *Stri Darpan*'s feminist persuasion and educative and reformist intent, both Ayurvedic and Western idioms of medicine were used to critique certain practices newly considered harmful to women. Medical arguments were used most prominently to condemn the institution of purdah, or female veiling and seclusion. As Janakdulari Gurtu argued,

> The reason that the health of the women of Hindustan is bad is because they do not get fresh air, because they stay closed inside purdah, the movement of all of the limbs of their body is minimal, and fresh air does not reach their lungs. Tuberculosis, anemia, etc. very many diseases catch hold of their *palle* [ends of their saris].[77]

Research conducted by British and Indian women physicians in the late 1910s and 1920s had begun documenting high rates of infant and maternal mortality, tuberculosis, and osteomalacia among Indian women, linking incidence to the purdah system and to the ill effects of early marriage and sexual intercourse.[78] *Stri Darpan* reflected these growing concerns by publishing articles on tuberculosis and women in India that connected it with purdah.[79] Other authors utilized medical arguments to argue for the reform of child marriage, viewing the custom as a leading social evil that compromised India's standing in the world community:

> The increasing infant mortality rate, the death of countless girl-mothers during their pregnancies or at childbirth, the spread of various new diseases in the offspring of these girl-mothers if saved from death, the decreasing life expectancy of our country's inhabitants, and the downward decline of our bodily, spiritual, and mental condition – all this is the fruit of this degraded custom of child marriage. Is there any other country in the world apart from Hindustan where one could find widows of one year or less? We are forced to lower our head in front of the world's civilized nations/races for these very reasons.[80]

Weakness and physical debility were also criticized as characteristics of Indian women that needed reform. Authors emphasized that exercise should be performed regularly by women, notwithstanding their own feelings of shame and the criticisms of traditionalists who considered it a masculine practice. As K. N. Tandon noted in an article on the importance of health and health maintenance, "Nowadays, for women, to exercise is considered a matter of great shame; [people ask] is it that women want to become wrestlers that they need to exercise?" Tandon responded,

> If doing exercise is a matter of embarrassment, then is it that being weak is a matter of great fortune and an adornment to women? What element of embarrassment is there in doing that by which we can make and keep our health, beauty, etc., everything, in short, and also fulfill our hopes of seeing our children strong and free of disease?[81]

Thus the ideal future female citizen being promoted in journals such as *Stri Darpan* was one fashioned by knitting together older ideals with newer goals: a reformed, cultured woman; assumed to be middle-class and upper-caste; educated in the Ayurvedic and Western hygienic traditions; knowledgeable about an older cultural (and implicitly Hindu) heritage from which she could extract elements of value without being blindly beholden to tradition; unrestricted by earlier forms of seclusion and modesty yet not too Westernized in habit and comportment; and remaining ultimately a respectable and self-sacrificing mother and wife. Endowed with new responsibilities and allowed certain new privileges and freedoms, she was simultaneously subject to novel demands and constraints.

Indeed, similar ideals and practices were already being promoted in other parts of India, as a number of historians have shown, most notably in Bengal and Punjab.[82] In Punjab, in the new vernacular language schools established by the Hindu reformist organization the Arya Samaj, girls were instructed to write letters describing disease symptoms to a physician, and domestic economy, nursing, and hygiene were considered important subjects in the curriculum. As Madhu Kishwar has argued, one of the main purposes of the Kanya Mahavidyalaya (Girls' High Schools) was to produce the "modern" housewife, and lessons on nutrition, scientific causes of disease, and methods of nursing invalids and children were viewed as essential for doing so. Because Arya ideology stressed that the primary role of women was to reproduce the race, women's own health also became a central concern for those advocating "race maintenance." Such concerns focused on women's lack of physical exercise and exposure to fresh air, and their ignorance of proper food habits, seen as a primary cause of disease.[83]

Similarly, in late nineteenth century Bengal, as Dipesh Chakrabarty has argued, health and hygiene became important components of a nationalist civilizing discourse that attempted to refashion such disciplines of bodily practice as eating habits and care of children and the sick. Derived from a colonial critique of indigenous practices, this discourse was primarily intended for the Bengali middle-class housewife, attempting to reform her values and behavior to bring them into closer alignment with the changing demands of the newly constituted colonial bourgeois public sphere. Along with this "civilizing" discourse, Chakrabarty argues, Bengali modernity also consisted of what he calls a "dharmic discourse." This idiom, predicated on the "difference" that nationalism required, refurbished an older patriarchal ideal that centered on the Hindu goddess Lakshmi. No less dependent on education, such an ideal insisted however that too much education would create Alakshmis (anti-Lakshmis); traditional feminine values of grace and modesty were stressed to ideally produce the modern yet fully national Bengali woman.[84]

While Kishwar's and Chakrabarty's analyses have been important models for my own approach to similar source materials, they and other historians of colonial India have tended to overlook the specific and changing content of conceptions such as "hygiene" and "medicine." "Hygiene" in such accounts has occupied a kind of ahistorical space, one that requires no investigation on its own terms as a category with changing referents; its genealogy has been seen as unproblematic. I would suggest rather that the use of such terms served as nodes around which an array of meanings and identities clustered, but which varied according to particular local and historical contexts. To read such tropes flatly, as indicative only of a Western, modernizing discourse, is to miss the historical complexity and malleability of the terms' referents. As I have demonstrated, hygiene – understood as prevention of disease and preservation and promotion of health, was not simply a sign of a "civilizing" Western discourse but was also deeply central to Ayurvedic discourse.[85] Similarly, much of the secondary literature that has examined the increased concern about childcare and maternal health in early twentieth-century India has not addressed what I have identified as a partnership and tension between Ayurvedic and biomedically derived notions of health and the body. Scholars have seen arguments for reform as derived solely from Western medicine, reflecting the hegemony of Western medicine within female nationalist discourse.[86] My analysis stresses that among a Hindi vernacular élite, Western medicine had far from established a monolithic hegemony by the 1920s. Furthermore, I suggest that without close attention to the specific and changing historical meanings associated with medical terms and practices, we cannot fully understand the nature of the complex, often contradictory and ambivalent processes by which Western medicine has been able to extend its hold over larger portions of the world's populations, while often being unable to fully supplant differing medical traditions.

Conclusion

When *Stri Darpan* began publication in 1909, Western medical knowledge and practice had circulated in India for some centuries. Having contributed to the constitution of British and European superiority during the age of imperialism, Western medicine did also influence the identities of certain Indian social groups. For many *Stri Darpan* authors, Western medicine had enormous impact, redefining their conceptions of themselves and their bodily capacities. Humiliated in the face of British criticism and convinced that ameliorating India's situation required urgent action, many *Stri Darpan* authors took on high infant mortality rates, negligent childcare practices, and the negative health effects of social customs such as purdah and child marriage as their own national problems.

At the same time, it is clear that Western medicine had not become the hegemonic medical framework among the regional north Indian élite that comprised the audience for journals such as *Stri Darpan*. *Stri Darpan* itself advocated an implicitly dual medicine, one which promoted the appreciation, use, and knowledge of a revitalized Ayurveda in addition to accepting aspects of the Western medical model. *Stri Darpan* seemed to suggest that the Indian nation could accommodate – indeed, required – both the Western and Ayurvedic medical traditions, despite significant differences in their conceptions of the body, disease definitions and etiologies, and understandings about health. *Stri Darpan* authors and readers thus linked the pursuit of modernity with a simultaneous search for origins and authenticity – seen as essential characteristics of a national identity – so that the would-be modern Indian nation could possess a venerable pedigree. The *Stri Darpan* resolution consisted of a selective appropriation of Western medical knowledge while contesting colonial hegemony, selective reformation of indigenous practices identified as outmoded, and a revaluation and revitalization of Ayurvedic medicine, which was seen as authentic, ancient, and indigenous.[87]

Due to their cultural and historical associations, medical traditions often function as important symbols, even as expressions of national identity and pride. Yet medicine also serves to define identities through its status as a moral, prescriptive discourse. As we have seen, both Western and Ayurvedic medical idioms were used to shape certain new kinds of Indian women, to alter their relationships to their bodies and the bodies of their families. Cast as mothers of the nation, reproducers and nurturers of its future generations, Indian women became the focus of anxieties centered on national viability and the target of intensive reform efforts that struck at the very heart of the domestic realm, yet linked that realm to wider communities and identities. *Stri Darpan* therefore also illustrates the extent to which medical conceptions can be influential in elaborating new gender, class, caste, religious, and national identities. The malleable discourses of health and medicine operated at a prescriptive level, with implications for individual behavior, community regulation, and social policy. The small but growing number of newly literate middle-class, upper-caste north Indian women who read *Stri Darpan* were tutored to assume the weight of their responsibilities to the future Indian nation, responsibilities that sought to govern literally their bodies and those of their families as well as shape their minds.

Acknowledgment

I would like to thank David Arnold, Amrit Gahunia, Henrika Kuklick, Donna Mehos, Kapil Raj, Charles Rosenberg, Dominik Wujastyk, and especially Molly Sutphen and Bridie Andrews for their comments and suggestions at various points in this chapter's evolution.

Notes

1. Doctor Shrikant Tripathi, "*Bacce Kyoṁ Marte Haiṁ*" [Why Do Children Die?], *Stri Darpan* 29:6 (June 1923): 648, 651. All translations from the Hindi are my own. "National crime" was written in English.
2. [Rameshwari Nehru], "*Prāṇāyām aur Deśī Kasrat*" [Pranayam and National Exercise], *Stri Darpan* 20:2 (Feb. 1919): 61.
3. Dominik Wujastyk, "Indian Medicine," in *Companion Encyclopedia of the History of Medicine*, eds W. F. Bynum and Roy Porter (London: Routledge, 1993), 767, 770–1; Kenneth G. Zysk, *Asceticism and Healing in Ancient India: Medicine in the Buddhist Monastery* (Delhi: Oxford University Press, 1991); M. N. Pearson, "The Thin End of the Wedge: Medical Relativities as a Paradigm of Early Modern Indian-European Relations," *Modern Asian Studies* 29:1 (1995): 168–9; Mark Harrison, *Public Health in British India: Anglo-Indian Preventive Medicine 1859–1914* (Cambridge: Cambridge University Press, 1994), 7. See Dominik Wujastyk, *The Roots of Ayurveda: Selections from Sanskrit Medical Writings* (New Delhi: Penguin, 1998), for an accessible introduction to classical Ayurvedic thought. An Ayurvedic physician is known as a *vaid* or *vaidya*. A *hakām* is a physician who practices Unani medicine.
4. These remarks refer primarily to the colonies with large non-European populations. See the following for a small selection of the early works in this rapidly growing field: David Arnold, *Colonizing the Body: State Medicine and Epidemic Disease in Nineteenth-Century India* (Berkeley: University of California Press, 1993); ibid., "Medicine and Colonialism," in *Companion Encyclopedia of the History of Medicine*, eds W. F. Bynum and Roy Porter, vol. 2 (London:

Routledge, 1993), 1393–416; ibid., ed., *Imperial Medicine and Indigenous Societies* (Manchester: Manchester University Press, 1988); Andrew Cunningham and Bridie Andrews, eds, *Western Medicine as Contested Knowledge* (Manchester: Manchester University Press, 1997); Steven Feierman and John M. Janzen, eds, *The Social Basis of Health and Healing in Africa* (Berkeley: University of California Press, 1992); Harrison, *Public Health in British India*; Roy McLeod and Milton Lewis, eds, *Disease, Medicine, and Empire* (London: Routledge, 1988); Megan Vaughan, *Curing their Ills: Colonial Power and African Illness* (Cambridge: Polity Press, 1991).

5 This is not to ascribe a monolithic homogeneity to European identity or to Western medicine, but to acknowledge that historical actors themselves constructed such correlations. In practice, as Megan Vaughan has argued with reference to literature on healing in Africa, scientific medicine needs to be examined in its various forms and with greater attention to detail and historical context, not "reduced to its theory of itself" and placed in opposition to non-Western healing practices. See Megan Vaughan, "Healing and Curing: Issues in the Social History and Anthropology of Medicine in Africa," *Social History of Medicine* 7 (1994): 283–95.

6 See, for example, Arnold, *Colonizing the Body*, 244; Harrison, *Public Health in British India*, 1; Radhika Ramasubban, "Imperial Health in British India, 1857–1900," in *Disease, Medicine, and Empire*, eds, Roy MacLeod and Milton Lewis (London: Routledge, 1988), 38–60. Arnold argues, however, that Western medicine did gain increasing influence over the thoughts and behaviors of Indians, especially after 1914.

7 For recent work which takes up this task, see Deepak Kumar, "Unequal Contenders, Uneven Ground: Medical Encounters in British India, 1820–1920," in *Western Medicine as Contested Knowledge*, eds, Andrew Cunningham and Bridie Andrews (Manchester: Manchester University Press, 1997), 172–90; and several of the essays in Biswamoy Pati and Mark Harrison, eds, *Health, Medicine and Empire: Perspectives on Colonial India* (New Delhi: Orient Longman, 2001).

8 I am deeply indebted to Vir Bharat Talwar for directing me to extant copies of *Stri Darpan*.

9 See Benedict Anderson, *Imagined Communities: Reflections on the Origin and Spread of Nationalism*, 2nd edn (London: Verso, 1991 [orig. 1983]); E. J. Hobsbawm, *Nations and Nationalism Since 1780: Programme, Myth, Reality* (Cambridge: Cambridge University Press, 1990); Homi Bhabha, ed., *Nation and Narration* (London: Routledge, 1990); Stuart Hall, "Cultural Identity and Diaspora," in *Colonial Discourse and Post-Colonial Theory: A Reader*, eds, Patrick Williams and Laura Chrisman (Hertfordshire: Harvester Wheatsheaf, 1993), 392–403; and Geoff Eley and Ronald Grigor Suny, "Introduction: From the Moment of Social History to the Work of Cultural Representation," in *Becoming National: A Reader*, eds, Geoff Eley and Ronald Grigor Suny (New York: Oxford University Press, 1996), 6–8. The Eley and Suny reader provides an excellent introduction to the vast scholarship on nationalism.

10 Vir Bharat Talwar, "Feminist Consciousness in Women's Journals in Hindi: 1910–1920," in *Recasting Women: Essays in Colonial History*, eds, Kumkum Sangari and Sudesh Vaid (New Delhi: Kali for Women, 1989), 222–3; Francesca Orsini, "Domesticity and Beyond: Hindi Women's Journals in the Early Twentieth Century," *South Asia Research* 19:2 (1999): 138.

11 Purdah, literally "curtain" or "screen," is a shorthand term that has referred generally to the varied set of cultural practices, including the customs of veiling and seclusion, which aim to enforce high standards of female modesty and regulate relations between the sexes in many parts of South Asia. See Hanna Papanek and Gail Minault, "Foreword," in *Separate Worlds: Studies of Purdah*

in South Asia, eds, Hanna Papanek and Gail Minault (Columbia, MO: South Asia Books, 1982), vii–viii; and Hanna Papanek, "Purdah: Separate Worlds and Symbolic Shelter," in *Separate Worlds*, 3–53.
12 Gail Minault, "Urdu Women's Magazines in the Early Twentieth Century," *Manushi* 48 (Sept.–Oct. 1988): 2–9; Gail Minault, *Secluded Scholars: Women's Education and Muslim Social Reform in Colonial India* (Delhi: Oxford University Press, 1998), 110–22.
13 Addressed to Master Joe, Jawaharlal's nickname at the time, the letter was instead delivered to the school's headmaster (also named Joe), who, shocked at its seditious tone, sent a warning letter to Jawaharlal's father. Upon learning that it was Rameshwari who had written it, he wrote back, "I am intensely amused to hear that it was a charming young lady who defied the British Raj! Give her my kind regards, and say that I hope some day, when she knows us better, she will like us more!" Joseph Wood to M. Nehru, quoted in Om Prakash Paliwal, *Rameshwari Nehru: Patriot and Internationalist* (New Delhi: National Book Trust, 1986), pages between 10 and 11; and B. R. Nanda, *The Nehrus, Motilal and Jawaharlal* (London: Allen & Unwin, 1962), 83–4.
14 In 1923, *Stri Darpan* moved to Kanpur, to be edited by Sumati Devi and Phulkumari Mehrotra. See Orsini, "Domesticity and Beyond," 145.
15 See the fond description of Rameshwari *bhabhi* by Vijaya Lakshmi Pandit, Jawaharlal Nehru's sister, in her *The Scope of Happiness: A Personal Memoir* (New York: Crown, 1979), 31; *bhābhī* is the Hindi kin term to refer to one's elder brother's (or cousin brother's) wife. The quotation, "Rameshwari was my ideal of Indian womanhood," is attributed to Kulsum Sayani, an educational activist and Gandhian nationalist, who is quoted in Geraldine Forbes, *Women in Modern India* (New York: Cambridge University Press, 1996), 201; see also Kamaladevi Chattopadhyay, *Inner Recesses, Outer Spaces: Memoirs* (New Delhi: Navrang, 1986), 143. For references to Rameshwari Nehru's range of activities, which included association with the Delhi Women's League, an influential role in the national Women's India Association (WIA), which advocated female suffrage, and later involvement in peace and nuclear disarmament efforts, see Pandit, *The Scope of Happiness*, 61–2; Forbes, *Women in Modern India*, 87, 106, 206; Paliwal, *Rameshwari Nehru*; Aparna Basu, "The Role of Women in the Indian Struggle for Freedom," in *Indian Women: From Purdah to Modernity*, ed., B. R. Nanda (New Delhi: Radiant, 1990 [orig. 1976]), 22; and her obituary in *Times of India* (Nov. 9, 1966), 1.
16 Talwar, "Feminist Consciousness," 204.
17 Ibid., 207, 210.
18 Pandit, *The Scope of Happiness*, 31.
19 Orsini, "Domesticity and Beyond," 145.
20 See Orsini, "Domesticity and Beyond," 145.
21 Quoted in Orsini, "Domesticity and Beyond," 143–4. The quote was from a banner under the journal's title.
22 Talwar, "Feminist Consciousness," 208. For further analysis of Gandhi's attitudes concerning women, see Madhu Kishwar, "Women and Gandhi," *Economic and Political Weekly* 20 (Oct. 5 and Oct. 12, 1985): 1691–702, 1753–8; and Sujata Patel, "Construction and Reconstruction of Woman in Gandhi," *Economic and Political Weekly* 23 (Feb. 20, 1988): 377–87. The extent of *Stri Darpan*'s circulation is unclear, although Francesca Orsini argues that it remained relatively small, never more than 1,000 copies. While this may be true, there is considerable evidence that Indian newspapers and journals circulated much more widely, by, for example, being passed around to friends and relations or being read aloud in public, than their official figures would suggest.
23 Radha Kumar, *The History of Doing: An Illustrated Account of Movements for*

Women's Rights and Feminism in India, 1800–1990 (New Delhi: Kali for Women, 1993), 1.
24 Kumar, *The History of Doing*, 1.
25 The relation between the women's movement and the nationalist movement is complex and continues to be a subject of debate. See Geraldine Forbes, "The Politics of Respectability: Indian Women and the Indian National Congress," in *The Indian National Congress: Centenary Hindsights*, ed., D. A. Low (Delhi: Oxford University Press, 1988), 54–97; ibid., "The Women's Movement in India: Traditional Symbols and New Roles," in *Social Movements in India*, vol. 2, ed., M. S. A. Rao (Delhi: Manohar, 1979), 149–65; ibid., *Women in Modern India* (Cambridge: Cambridge University Press, 1996); Kumar, *The History of Doing*; and Susie Tharu and K. Lalita, eds, *Women Writing in India*, vol. I: 600 BC to the Early 20th Century (Delhi: Oxford University Press, 1993): 160–86.
26 The leading exponent of this view is Partha Chatterjee, "The Nationalist Resolution of the Women's Question," in *Recasting Women: Essays in Colonial History*, eds, Kumkum Sangari and Sudesh Vaid (New Delhi: Kali for Women, 1989), 233–54.
27 See Sonal Shukla, "Cultivating Minds: 19th Century Gujarati Women's Journals," *Economic and Political Weekly* 26:43 (Oct. 26, 1991): WS63–6; Orsini, "Domesticity and Beyond," 137–60.
28 Tharu and Lalita, *Women Writing in India*, 167.
29 Ibid., 167–70; Minault, "Urdu Women's Magazines," 2–9; Orsini, "Domesticity and Beyond," 137–60.
30 Rosalind O'Hanlon, *A Comparison Between Women and Men: Tarabai Shinde and the Critique of Gender Relations in Colonial India* (Madras: Oxford University Press, 1994), 38. See also Sumanta Banerjee, "Marginalization of Women's Popular Culture in Nineteenth Century Bengal," in *Recasting Women: Essays in Colonial History*, eds, Kumkum Sangari and Sudesh Vaid (New Delhi: Kali for Women, 1989), 127–79; Tharu and Lalita, *Women Writing in India*; and Minault, "Urdu Women's Magazines."
31 Alongside these were many other local varieties such as Avadhi, Bhojpuri, and Braj Bhasha.
32 This and the following three paragraphs are synthesized from R. S. McGregor, *Hindi Literature of the Nineteenth and Early Twentieth Centuries* (Wiesbaden: Otto Harrassowitz, 1974); Peter Gaeffke, *Hindi Literature in the Twentieth Century* (Wiesbaden: Otto Harrassowitz, 1978); David Lelyveld, "The Fate of Hindustani: Colonial Knowledge and the Project of a National Language," in *Orientalism and the Postcolonial Predicament: Perspectives on South Asia*, eds, Carol A. Breckenridge and Peter van der Veer (Philadelphia: University of Pennsylvania Press, 1993), 189–214; Krishna Kumar, "Quest for Self-Identity: Cultural Consciousness and Education in the Hindi Region, 1880–1950," *Economic and Political Weekly* 25:23 (June 9, 1990): 1247–9, 1251–5; Christopher King, *One Language, Two Scripts: The Hindi Movement in Nineteenth Century North India* (Bombay: Oxford University Press, 1994); C. A. Bayly, *Empire and Information: Intelligence Gathering and Social Communication in India, 1780–1870* (Cambridge: Cambridge University Press, 1996); and Francesca Orsini, "What Did They Mean by 'Public'? Language, Literature and the Politics of Nationalism," *Economic and Political Weekly* 34:7 (Feb. 13, 1999): 409–16.
33 Numerous books on Unani, Ayurvedic, and Western medicine and hygiene, including some translated from English, Persian, Arabic, and Sanskrit, were also being written and published in Urdu and Hindustani during the nineteenth and early twentieth centuries in northern India, from places such as Lahore, Lucknow, Kanpur, Agra, and Delhi. For example, T. H. Huxley's textbook of physiology was published in Lahore in 1877.

34 During the period from 1856–1910, almost 400 literary works, including plays, novels, essays, poems, and autobiographies, were written by almost 200 Bengali women authors. Twenty-one Bengali periodicals were edited by women and concerned themselves primarily with women's issues. See Banerjee, "Marginalization of Women's Popular Culture," 160. Meredith Borthwick has carefully detailed the importance attached to matters of hygiene and reformed childbirth and medical practices in this genre of Bengali literature. See Meredith Borthwick, *The Changing Role of Women in Bengal, 1849–1905* (Princeton, NJ: Princeton University Press, 1984).
35 Talwar, "Feminist Consciousness," 210.
36 See Eley and Suny, "Introduction," in *Becoming National*, 7.
37 Shrimati Prem Dulari, "*Khānā aur Uskā Tarīqā*" [How to Eat Food Properly], *Stri Darpan* 27:2 (Aug. 1922): 67; Shri Jagannath Shukla, "Dharmasàstra aur ārogyatà" [Dharmashastras and Health] *Stri Darpan* 27:2 (Aug. 1922): 72.
38 [Nehru], "*Prāṇāyām aur Deśī Kasrat*" [Pranayam and National Exercise], 61.
39 Dulari, "*Khānā aur Uskā Tarīqā*" [How to Eat Food Properly], 67–9; Shriyut B. K. Mitra, "*Ajīrṇ*" [Indigestion], *Stri Darpan* 16:5 (May 1917): 264.
40 Dulari, "*Khānā aur Uskā Tarīqā*" [How to Eat Food Properly], 67–9.
41 See Francis Zimmermann, "Rtu-Satmya: The Seasonal Cycle and the Principle of Appropriateness," *Social Science and Medicine* 14B (1980): 99–106.
42 *Asoj* (or *Āśvin*) and *Kārttik*, corresponding to 15 September–15 October and 15 October–15 November, respectively, are the seventh and eighth months of the Hindu lunar calendar. Dulari, "*Khānā aur Uskā Tarīqā*" [How to Eat Food Properly], 69. Cf. G. J. Meulenbeld, *The Madhavanidana and Its Chief Commentary* (Leiden: E. J. Brill, 1974), 449–50; and S. K. Ramachandra Rao, ed., *Encyclopaedia of Indian Medicine*, vol. 2 (Bombay: Popular Prakashan, 1987), 186–7.
43 Shriyut B. K. Mitra, "*Koṣṭh Vaddhatā yā Qabz*" [Constipation (or Contraction of Stomach)], *Stri Darpan* 16:6 (June 1917): 321–6; Mitra, "*Ajīrṇ*" [Indigestion], 262–7; Cf. Wujastyk, *The Roots of Ayurveda*, 5.
44 Mitra, "*Koṣṭh Vaddhatā yā Qabz*" [Constipation (or Contraction of Stomach)], 321–2.
45 See Sudhir Kakar, *Shamans, Mystics, and Doctors: A Psychological Inquiry into India and Its Healing Traditions* (Boston, MA: Beacon Press, 1982); and Francis Zimmermann, *The Jungle and the Aroma of Meats: An Ecological Theme in Hindu Medicine* (Berkeley, CA: University of California Press, 1987).
46 Shukla, "*Dharmaśāstra aur Ārogyatā*" [Dharmashastras and Health], 72–5.
47 Dulari, "*Khānā aur Uskā Tarīqā*" [How to Eat Food Properly], 69; Mitra, "*Ajīrṇ*" [Indigestion], 262–7; Shukla, "*Dharmaśāstra aur Ārogyatā*" [Dharmashastras and Health], 72.
48 [Nehru], "*Pustak Paricay*" [Book Conversation], 602.
49 "National crime" was written in English. See Tripathi, "*Bacce Kyoṁ Marte Haiṁ*" [Why Do Children Die?], 648, 651.
50 "Struggle for existence" and "Red Indians" were written in English; Shriyut Mukandilal, B.A. (Oxon.), Bar-at-Law, "*Śiśu Pālan*" [Childcare], *Stri Darpan* 23:3 (Sept. 1920): 117–20.
51 Doctor Prasadilal Jha, L.M.S., "*Acchī Dāiyoṁ kī Āvaśyaktā*" [The Need for Good Midwives], *Stri Darpan* 29:3 (Sept. 1923): 476–8; Mukandilal, "*Śiśu Pālan*" [Childcare], 117–20; Tripathi, "*Bacce Kyoṁ Marte Haiṁ*" [Why Do Children Die?], 647–51.
52 Tripathi, "*Bacce Kyoṁ Marte Haiṁ*" [Why Do Children Die?], 651.
53 Ibid., 649–50.
54 The allusion Tripathi used to describe the plight of the trapped man, that of the character Abhimanyu in the Hindu epic *Mahabharata*, is particularly

illuminating. Abhimanyu, son of the second Pandava brother Arjuna and his wife Subhadra, becomes trapped in the great war in a lotus configuration formed by the enemy Kauravas from which, despite fighting heroically, he is unable to escape. Tripathi, "*Bacce Kyoṁ Marte Haiṁ*" [Why Do Children Die?], 650.
55 Tripathi, "*Bacce Kyoṁ Marte Haiṁ*" [Why Do Children Die?], 650.
56 Jha, "*Acchī Dāiyoṁ kī Āvaśyaktā*" [The Need for Good Midwives], 477–8.
57 Janakdulari Gurtu, "*Tandurustī yānī Ārogyatā*" [Health or Absence of Illness], *Stri Darpan* 19:4 (Oct. 1918): 214.
58 [Nehru], "*Gaṅgājal se Svāsthya kī Hāni*" [Harm to Health from Ganges Water], *Stri Darpan* 20:1 (Jan. 1919): 6. The Hindi word used for "germ" was *kçmi*, which means "worm" or sometimes "small insect." It appears that *kçmi* was a term that was later infused with notions derived from the germ theory of disease of Western medicine, although this is a supposition that needs to be confirmed by further research. I gratefully acknowledge Dominik Wujastyk's discussions with me on this matter.
59 Jha, "*Acchī Dāiyoṁ kī Āvaśyaktā*" [The Need for Good Midwives], 476–8.
60 Tripathi, "*Bacce Kyoṁ Marte Haiṁ*" [Why Do Children Die?], 649; Jha, "*Acchī Dāiyoṁ kī Āvaśyaktā*" [The Need for Good Midwives], 476–8.
61 Charles Leslie, "Interpretations of Illness: Syncretism in Modern Ayurveda," in *Paths to Asian Medical Knowledge*, ed., Charles Leslie and Allan Young (Berkeley, CA: University of California Press, 1992), 177–208; ibid., "Ayurveda, Cosmopolitan Medicine, and Other Traditions in South Asia," in *Paths to Asian Medical Knowledge*, ed., Don Bates (Berkeley, CA: University of California Press, 1992), 128; Brahmananda Gupta, "Indigenous Medicine in Nineteenth and Twentieth-Century Bengal," in *Asian Medical Systems*, ed., Charles Leslie (Berkeley, CA: University of California Press, 1976), 368–77; Paul Brass, "The Politics of Ayurvedic Education: A Case Study of Revivalism and Modernization in India," in *Education and Politics in India*, eds, S. H. Rudolph and L. I. Rudolph (Cambridge, MA: Harvard University Press, 1972), 342–71, 452–9; K. N. Panikkar, "Indigenous Medicine and Cultural Hegemony: A Study of the Revitalization Movement in Keralam," *Studies in History* 8:2 (1992): 283–308; Poonam Bala, *Imperialism and Medicine in Bengal: A Socio-historical Perspective* (New Delhi: Sage, 1991); Harrison, *Public Health in British India*.
62 Ibid.
63 Dulari, "*Khāṇā aur Uskā Tarīqā*" [Food and Its Proper Method], 67–8.
64 Sundarimohan Das, "Resurrection of Motherhood and Fatherhood," *Modern Review* 26:2 (Aug. 1919): 189–92; excerpted, translated, and reprinted as "*Mātā kā Navjīvan*" [New Life for Mother] in *Stri Darpan* 21:5 (Nov. 1919): 239–41.
65 Occasionally *hamārī jāti* (our community, subcaste) or *hamārā yahāṁ* (literally "our here, place") were also used. See Mukandilal, "*Śiśu Pālan*" [Childcare], 118–20; Vishvanath Prasad Mishra, "*Śiśu Pālan Rahasya*" [Secrets of Childcare], *Stri Darpan* 27:5 (Nov. 1922): 242–5; Dulari, "*Khāṇā aur Uskā Tarīqā*" [Food and its Proper Method], 67–9; Jha, "*Acchī Dāiyoṁ kī Āvaśyaktā*" [Need for Good Midwives], 476–8.
66 Dipesh Chakrabarty, "The Difference/Deferral of (A) Colonial Modernity: Public Debates on Domesticity in British Bengal," *History Workshop* 36 (1993): 6.
67 Dulari, "*Khāṇā aur Uskā Tarīqā*" [Food and its Proper Method], 68.
68 [Nehru], "*Pustak Paricay*" [Book Conversation], 602.
69 "*Śiśu Pālan meṁ Kuch Zarūrī Bāteṁ*" [Some Necessary Points Concerning Childcare], *Stri Darpan* 29:2 (Aug. 1923): 396–7. In this article, doctors and vaids were classed as equivalent medical authorities. See also Mukandilal, "*Śiśu Pālan*" [Childcare], 117–20.
70 Chatterjee, "Nationalist Resolution of the Women's Question," 240–9.

71 Mitra, "*Koṣṭh Vaddhatā yā Qabz*" [Constipation (or Contraction of Stomach)], 321–6.
72 Shri Mukutvihari Lal Dar, "*Bhārat meṁ Kṣay Rog aur Striyāṁ*" [Tuberculosis and Women in India], *Stri Darpan* 22:1 (Jan. 1920): 29.
73 Doctor Mahendralal Garg, "*Acchā Putr Pāne kā Upāy*" [Means to Obtain a Good Son], *Stri Darpan* 21:3 (Sept. 1919): 143–4. The Puranas are sacred texts of Hinduism that consist of religious instruction as well as genealogies and legends of gods and royal dynasties. The Matsya Purana (*matsya*, literally fish, refers to one of the avatars of Vishnu) is considered one of the eighteen major Puranas.
74 Mitra, "*Ajīrṇ*" [Indigestion], 262.
75 Jha, "*Acchī Dāiyoṁ kī Āvaśyaktā*" [Need for Good Midwives], 476.
76 For reference to healing practice among Muslim women that was denigrated by reformers promoting a revitalized Unani medical tradition, see Barbara Metcalf, *Perfecting Women: Maulana Ashraf'Ali Thanawi's "Bihisti Zewar": Partial Translation and Commentary* (Delhi: Oxford University Press, 1990), 10. However, it would be unwise to romanticize women's access to and control of medical and healing knowledge in earlier times. Ayurvedic medicine, for instance, offered no place to women healers; in Dominik Wujastyk's words, its "gaze remain[ed] unwaveringly male." See Wujastyk, *Roots of Ayurveda*, 23. Nevertheless, Wujastyk has stressed in personal communication that Ayurvedic literature did contain "quite a lot of instruction and description . . . about women's bodies and the treatment of female conditions."
77 Gurtu, "*Tandurustī yānī Ārogyatā*" [Health or Absence of Illness], 214.
78 For more detailed analysis of the medical research linking purdah to disease and its circulation in wider social contexts, see my article, "Purdah as Pathology: Gender and the Circulation of Medical Knowledge in Late Colonial India," forthcoming in *Rocking the Cradle: Essays in India's Reproductive History*, ed. Sarah Hodges (New Delhi: Permanent Black).
79 Dar, "*Bhārat meṁ Kṣay Rog aur Striyāṁ*" [Tuberculosis and Women in India], 25–31.
80 Shrimati Vidyavati Khanna, "*Bāl Vivāh aur Usse Jātī kā Hāniyāṁ*" [Child Marriage and its Harmfulness to Society], *Stri Darpan* 22:5 (May 1920): 276.
81 K. N. Tandon, "*Ārogyatā*" [Health], *Stri Darpan* 17:4 (Oct. 1917): 198–9.
82 Chakrabarty, "Difference/Deferral of (A) Colonial Modernity"; Samita Sen, "Motherhood and Mothercraft: Gender and Nationalism in Bengal," *Gender and History* 5:2 (1993): 231–43; and Madhu Kishwar, "Arya Samaj and Women's Education: Kanya Mahavidyalaya, Jalandhar," *Economic and Political Weekly* 21:17 (Apr. 26, 1986): WS9–WS24.
83 *Panchal Pandita*, "solely devoted to interests of Indian women," was started in 1897 as the monthly organ of the Kanya Mahavidyalaya. See Madhu Kishwar, "Daughters of Aryavarta," *Indian Economic and Social History Review* 23 (1986): 108–9; ibid., "Arya Samaj and Women's Education," WS12–WS15.
84 Chakrabarty, "Difference/Deferral of (A) Colonial Modernity."
85 The fact that Chakrabarty focuses on the discourse of health and hygiene only in his discussion of the "civilizing" discourse, with medical or hygienic concepts not referred to in his description of Bengali "dharmic" discourse, points to the lack of symmetry in his treatment of these two idioms.
86 Cf., for example, Sen, "Motherhood and Mothercraft."
87 Cf. Partha Chatterjee, *The Nation and Its Fragments: Colonial and Postcolonial Histories* (Princeton, NJ: Princeton University Press, 1993). It is likely no accident that *Stri Darpan* promoted Ayurveda, long associated with Hinduism, rather than Unani medicine, associated with Islam, for its revitalization project.

3 A sword of empire?
Medicine and colonialism at King William's Town, Xhosaland, 1856–91

David Gordon

Introduction

One evening in 1856 a renowned Xhosa doctor (or *igqirha*), Gota, while suffering from sore eyes, dreamt that someone burnt him on the forehead. The assailant then turned to Gota's brother-in-law, the long-deceased King Ngqika, and attempted to burn him. Ngqika escaped, but before disappearing told Gota to seek relief at the house of a white doctor sent by the Queen of England. The next morning Gota considered the meaning of his dream and decided to heed the advice of the dead King Ngqika. Gota set off to consult the European doctor. After a few days travel he arrived in King William's Town, the frontier capital of the new colony called British Kaffraria (1847–65) where he went to the dispensary of the newly-appointed head of the Medical Department of British Kaffraria and Superintendent of Native Hospitals, Dr John Patrick Fitzgerald.[1]

Gota's experience was not exceptional. In the few months since Fitzgerald's arrival in King William's Town, many Xhosa[2] had sought therapy at the hospital provided by the Queen of England.[3] By May, after only two months, Fitzgerald could boast that the

> natives are coming to me from all directions.... [they] place an unlimited confidence in me and are to me in my professional capacity as obedient children.... I fear that like many kind friends among the Europeans they overestimate my services, but ... for zeal and devotion I will yield to none.[4]

In spite of Fitzgerald's seemingly benign intentions, colonial medical services at King William's Town were entwined in a web of political and cultural intrigues. Sir George Grey, the governor of the Cape from 1854 to 1861 (British Kaffraria fell under the jurisdiction of the Cape governor), established the King William's Town Hospital in the hope of transferring responsibility for healing from the rebellious and powerful African healers, called *amagqirha*, to a corps of European or European-trained doctors loyal to imperial authority.[5] Colonial intentions and actual outcomes often diverged, however. Grey's scheme failed, for, as Jeff Peires has perceptively noted in passing, "the Xhosa were able to swallow Fitzgerald's medicine without in any way giving up their beliefs in the powers in Xhosa doctors," and thus "the great contest between science and superstition which Grey had envisaged never occurred."[6] Indeed, the early years of the hospital point to the success of Africans in attaining medical benefits without the accouterments of colonial power, which many historians, trusting the devious discourse of characters like Sir George Grey, have believed to be inextricably bound together.[7]

David Arnold has acknowledged that colonial medicine was not an obvious hegemonic instrument:

> The colonizing force of Western medicine has to be understood as more than a crude device of imperial self-legitimation, a mere "tool of empire." Medicine also marked out a ragged arena full of unresolved issues, a contested space as well as a colonizing one. . . . It [Western medicine] had to fashion its own compromise, negotiate its own passage, between the laws laid down in the scientific metropolis and the practical possibilities and priorities determined by colonial rule over an "alien" society.[8]

The story that this chapter tells is not one of Western doctors colonizing African bodies, but of the vicissitudes of an encounter between Europeans and Africans struggling to control knowledge and resources of healing techniques in the context of changing political alignments. At first the weak colonial state and the nature of pre-capitalist settler encroachment allowed for an important exchange of medical ideas and identities, leading to a dynamic therapeutic pluralism. The very distinctions between "European" and "African," or "modern" and "traditional," medicine began to collapse as the "quest for therapy" – as medical anthropologist John Janzen described the process in his classic work – helped to create a peculiar medical culture.[9] Africans could accept the beneficial aspects of this colonial medicine without conceding their central ideas about the nature of healing. Colonial medicine was also transformed as Fitzgerald began to accept and incorporate different African medical practices.

Increasingly, however, as settler power grew and state institutions solidified, little room was left for cultural interchange of any form. With the complete victory of settler forces over the southern Nguni polities and the beginnings of proletarianization in response to the rise of the mining industry, the avenues for collaboration between European and African cultures narrowed.[10] In the late nineteenth century the germ theory grounded Western medicine in a new scientific therapeutics that disdained "supersitions" of the past and had less respect for alternative therapeutic systems.[11] Colonial medicine became embroiled in a new "modernizing" project that constructed African medicine as its "primitive" Other. Local medical institutions fell under the stricter institutional control of the local Cape government, or, more precisely, the ominous-sounding Supreme Medical Committee. African healers were denounced, funding for African hospitals was reduced, and African patients lost their ability to control and guide their therapeutic quest.

Siyavuma: building consent

Prior to the arrival of European medicine, a variety of African healing practices flourished. Oral and ethnographic evidence indicates the broad traditions to which Xhosa medicine belonged; more specific details need to be gleaned from European accounts of actual medical practices in nineteenth-century Xhosaland. Fortunately, we have an informative manuscript written by Dr Fitzgerald who was fascinated by the African healing traditions (even though he was sure of the superiority of European medicine). The manuscript details the therapy of three "opthalmia" patients who underwent a total of twenty-four different consultations before they came to be treated at the hospital.[12] Combined with more recent ethnographic accounts, it enables us to reconstruct some of the features of Xhosa medical culture in the mid-nineteenth century.

Xhosa medicine was a variation of the widespread medical institution that Western anthropologists have named "cult of affliction" or "ngoma" (meaning drum or dance in many Bantu languages).[13] The Xhosa believed that sickness was an attempt at communication by ancestral spirits and to understand the reason for this communication, the Xhosa sufferer, accompanied by friends or family, would visit an *igqirha*.[14] As soon as this therapy group arrived, the *igqirha* proceeded to divine the reason for the visit and diagnose the disease. As the *igqirha* mouthed the divinations revealed by the ancestors, the visiting company would beat a drum and chant *Siyavuma* (we agree or we consent).[15] The ritual varied in its elaboration; sometimes sacrifices of goats and cattle, feasts, and dances were necessary before the ancestors revealed their will. Nevertheless, the divination (or diagnosis) was an attempt at a consensus between the voices of the ancestors spoken through the *igqirha* on the one hand and the therapy group on the other.

Yet the therapeutic quest was often complicated and could involve several intermediaries. Of the twenty-four consultations in Fitzgerald's three case studies, six were simply dealt with by herbalists, three were attributed to curses, six to ancestral wrath and eleven to a calling to become an *igqirha*.[16] The herbalists (or *amaxhwele*), often women, were not concerned with the typical ancestral *ngoma* rituals. They administered plants and herbs which had a known therapeutic effect. This was often the first stage in a therapeutic quest.

If the herbalists failed to find a remedy, the sick turned to more complicated forms of "ngoma" therapy. In the three cases of curses, sickness was thought to be caused by a living person – a "witch" – and carried out through certain spirits. In a few rare cases this led to the consultation of a second type of doctor, an *igqirha elinukayo*, who then smelt out the person responsible for the curse (this did not happen in any of the three cases cited by Fitzgerald). If such an avenue were followed, those identified as witches may have been tortured, often to death, to force them to reveal the poison or fetish they had used to bewitch the sufferer. But such happenings were rare and usually only occurrred during times of great upheaval like European conquest or the onset of a previously unknown epidemic. In spite of the rarity of vengeance against witches, Sir George Grey cited cases of horrific torture – alleged witches being placed across red hot coals and slowly burnt – to make a case against African medicine and the *amagqirha* in general.[17]

More often bewitched patients would simply go to an *igqirha eliqubulayo* who then "sucked" out the bewitching matter. Instead of identifying other people responsible for misfortunes, the *igqirha* told his or her patients that ancestral wrath was responsible for their condition or that they had simply been bewitched or "eaten" by the spirit in the river. The prescription in these cases was to sacrifice cattle to propitiate the ancestors, or to throw certain medicines into the river.[18]

The most frequent diagnosis was that the sickness signified that the patient needed to accept his sickness and become an *igqirha*. The sick person needed "to come out" and accept his or her sickness. The Xhosa infinitive *ukuthwasa* – "to become visible" – is used to express the emergence of a sick person and an *umthwasisi* was the name of the *igqirha* who "brings out" the sickness. This "coming out" and acceptance would generally take place in a dream of a plant or animal, which would then become the healing symbol of the patient-doctor. Consent to sickness, and thus to the particular calling through a dream, was the first step towards purification and eventually to becoming a fully-fledged *igqirha*. The central concept of Xhosa medicine was thus consent (*vuma*) to the illness and to becoming an *igqirha* within a particular cult of affliction. After this acceptance, the patient-initiate paid the *igqirha* with goods that ranged from assegais to beads and money. Then the *igqirha* began treatment, including daily cleansing and the application of a variety of medicines. During this period of healing and initiation, which could last a few months, the patient-initiate would learn the secrets of healing. The efficacy of this healing process was of central importance, for an *igqirha* could only successfully recruit patient-initiates if the sufferers were satisfied that their condition had ameliorated. When the remedies of the *amagqirha* were believed to have failed, the patients demanded, often succesfully, that their initial payment be reimbursed.[19]

Through the consensual "cult of affliction," Xhosa medical culture extended beyond patient and doctor to include ancestors and kin in what John Janzen terms a "therapy group."[20] Consensus within this group over the cause of the disease was crucial to the initiation of healing. The group identified the living or dead human agent responsible for the misfortune and decided on the application of suitable measures to remedy the situation.

Healing thereby involved both social and physical realms. By doing so, it allowed the Xhosa, who could not rely on written records, to incorporate new therapeutic technologies and retain old ones.[21]

Dr John Patrick Fitzgerald came from a tradition in which the therapeutic strategies of the ancestors were inscribed in sacred, written texts and not oral traditions. A young Irish Catholic, Fitzgerald graduated at 25 from Glasgow in 1839 after specializing in opthalmics and maternal care. He immediately left for New Zealand to offer medical care to the Maori. New Zealand settlers opposed Fitzgerald, although imperial sponsorship enabled him to practice and by 1841 he reported a successful amputation of one Maori's arm which had "enhanced the confidence of local Maoris in European medical skill."[22] Sir George Grey, Governor of New Zealand from 1845 to 1854, encouraged his work. In the longer term, however, Fitzgerald's medical mission was hampered by conflict between settlers and the imperial government, anti-Catholic sentiment, and the demographic collapse of the Maori people in the face of epidemic smallpox against which Fitzgerald struggled in vain. Finally, the death of his young wife in 1852, followed by an attack of cholera, destroyed the young doctor; he resigned his post in the colonial medical service and returned to England in 1854.[23]

Fitzgerald's New Zealand experience proved to be an important political training ground for the role he later played in British Kaffraria. His skill in manipulating the imperial government through patrons like George Grey to achieve his medical goals was essential to the early success of the King William's Town Hospital. Fitzgerald secured the appointment of the head of the medical department and superintendent of the Native Hospital through Grey who had been transferred to British Kaffraria from New Zealand in 1854 (some evidence even suggests that Fitzgerald's move from New Zealand might have been planned by Grey and Fitzgerald before they left New Zealand).[24]

For Grey, the hospital was one in an array of colonial institutions which would demonstrate the benefits of European rule to the Xhosa. More precisely, he hoped it would weaken the resistance of the Xhosa to colonial rule. After Xhosa military defeat in 1853, Grey set about eroding traditional networks of political patronage by establishing institutions like the hospital which would destroy the power of the recalcitrant portion of the Xhosa élite. While Fitzgerald's personal correspondence indicates his sincere belief in a "benign" vision of curing the African sick, he also shared Grey's "civilizing mission" (although without its more ruthless imperial designs). It was the continued alliance between Grey's colonial ambitions and Fitzgerald's medical zeal, expressed in terms of a medical "civilizing mission", that formed the political backbone of the King William's Town Hospital. According to Fitzgerald's correspondence, Grey would sing the praise: "Grey is great and Fitzgerald is his witchdoctor."[25]

Fitzgerald launched into his "civilizing mission" by spreading his medicine, which he hoped would eliminate disease and thereby demonstrate the benefits of colonial rule. Soon after his arrival in March 1856, he wrote Colonel John Maclean, Chief Commissioner of British Kaffraria until 1864:

> I have been on horse back through the country a great deal attending to sick Natives and every where the Natives have hailed me with delight and have expressed themselves grateful to the Government for having sent me amongst them ... before ten years pass over many a savage heart will be won over to the British Government and many a Father and Mother or Husband and Wife will bless the benevolence and wisdom of that Government which entered in spirit into the sickness and sufferings of the black savage lying neglected and forlorn on the cold damp ground and suggested a remedy.[26]

The success of the benevolent mission was supposedly proved by a letter sent from a "Kaffir," M'toni Mohlati, to Queen Victoria, thanking her for sending Fitzgerald who restored his sight after a blindness of 16 years.[27] Yet despite the grand ideals and great plans, the transformative powers of Fitzgerald's medical mission were limited. Fitzgerald's form of medicine could not be imposed upon a *tabula rasa*; instead it had to be incorporated into existing medical traditions. This would make Fitzgerald's form of healing, like Christianity, a sword of empire that cut both ways.

The Xhosa had developed their own responses to the crushing events of the early 1850s. Besides defeat in 1853 which led to the traumatic implementation of colonial rule, a deadly bovine disease called lungsickness arrived from Europe. Although the effects were unevenly spread across the countryside, lungsickness killed about 5,000 cattle per month.[28] These catastrophic times engendered a number of healers and prophets who attempted to help the Xhosa understand and deal with the micro and macroparasitic plagues that swept across the land. These healers heard the cries of dead warriors, appealing for a purification which would lead to their resurrection; they initiated movements which tried to restore order to disintegrating political and ecological relationships. The most widespread and popular reaction was the Cattle-Killing inspired by the Prophetess Nongqawuse. In brief, between the middle of 1856 and 1857, a number of prophets instructed all cattle to be killed and crops destroyed. This would allow for the resurrection of all past warrior-ancestors and their cattle which had died from the lungsickness epizootic. The ancestors disappointed the Xhosa and the movement only contributed to famine and the further erosion of Xhosa independence.[29]

Fitzgerald arrived in Xhosaland several months before the Cattle-Killing prophecies. It seems that the Xhosa greeted the European healer in a similar fashion to the Prophetess Nongqawuse: he promised a new form of healing to deal with the catastrophic effects that the arrival of the colonists had for Xhosa society. For the first month that records were kept, May 1856, 940 men, women, and children traveled to the dispensary with a variety of complaints: respiratory problems, syphilis, skin ailments, and minor injuries.

At first, judging by the number of unidentifiable minor ailments, many wanted to simply be handled by this white doctor sent by the Queen of England. After the Cattle-Killing episode, however, numbers would drop dramatically (see Figure 3.1 on page 52).[30]

The reasons for Fitzgerald's initial success were twofold. First, his skill in performing minor surgical operations and in particular the removal of cataracts, which restored sight to the partially blind. Second, not unrelated to the first, Fitzgerald became known as a powerful magician. There were rumors that he only had to cut the strings of one girl's eyes to restore her sight and ensure a successful marriage. Others claimed that they had their youth restored. Fitzgerald's equipment inspired amazement – his glass cupping machine was thought to bleed only on his secret instructions and left no wound.[31] The Xhosa wanted to incorporate and develop the practical promises of Fitzgerald's new form of therapy.

What Grey did not realize was that the essence of the Fitzgerald medical mission's success was in this purification of so-called "science" by "superstition." Some interesting linguistic evidence illuminates this phenomenon. The name for opthalmia in Xhosa is *imvuma*, based on the verb *-vuma* (to agree or consent), which was the chant of the therapy group in response to the divination of the *igqirha*.[32] When patients arrived to be treated for opthalmia at Fitzgerald's dispensary, they consented to their illness and thereby to treatment by the new *igqirha* who was incorporated into existing medical cosmology. Usually Bantu languages have different nouns for African "traditional" and "modern" doctors. For example, in Zulu, an African doctor is an *inyanga* while a "modern" doctor is *udoktela* after the English "doctor." Yet in Xhosa the same noun *-gqirha* is used for "modern" and "traditional" doctors, although placed in different noun classes. European doctors became known as *ugqirha* (pl. *bagqirha*).[33]

There is nothing too surprising about the fact that the Xhosa believed that Fitzgerald performed healing miracles. A little more unexpected, however, was the ease and willingness with which the Xhosa incorporated new therapeutic technologies into their existing beliefs. Robin Horton provides a broader perspective to this phenomenon in his classic and widely-discussed essay which details the way in which "traditional" philosophers adopt and adapt modern knowledge:

> Now although the philosophers fill a thoroughly traditional role, the very nature of their involvement with the old cosmology makes it likely that they will be more acutely aware of the interpretive challenge of modern change than anyone else. Some will react by trying to deny change or campaigning for its reversal. Others, seeing that what has happened can neither be denied nor reversed, will set to work extending and developing the existing cosmology in such a way as to account for the new social situation and bring it under some sort of control. Hence, even if this new situation does not impinge very directly on their own

daily lives, they may be deeply involved with the new developments in cosmology and ritual, and may even take the lead in formulating such developments. Among the adherents of the new-style cosmology, then, we shall find not only a great many people obviously committed to a "modern" life, but also a handful who are drawn from the heart of the pre-modern world. We may even find the moderns being led by the pre-moderns.[34]

Rather than undermine the "traditional" *amagqirha* doctors, African healers were the first to greet Fitzgerald's medicine and mold it to existing medical cosmologies and cultural identities. They were eager to learn of the new technologies offered by Western medicine. As Franz Fanon has observed in his astute polemic against the effects of colonial medicine, those "who take destiny into their own hands assimilate the most modern forms of technology at an extraordinary rate."[35]

Gota, the great Xhosa doctor who dreamt of Fitzgerald, was one such healer. Through the dream of Fitzgerald, Gota consented to his illness and to a process of healing and initiation into Fitzgerald's medicine. After being treated, Gota and two companions stayed for the evening and discussed medical matters. They all exchanged therapies and talked of the variety of patients whom they had cured – Fitzgerald of the Maoris and Gota of the Europeans.[36] On Gota's departure, Fitzgerald told the *igqirha* to treat him as a friend, and Gota expressed his appreciation for "now I have a friend in Kaffir Land to whom I can come. . . . My heart is happy. I shall have a nice sleep."[37] Once initiated into Fitzgerald's "cult of affliction," Ngqika's ancestral spirit would protect Gota's nights. Gota maintained contact with Fitzgerald and often stayed at the hospital where he carefully observed Fitzgerald treating his patients.[38] Another *igqirha*, after spending a week in Fitzgerald's hospital, boasted that "I shall have my Kraal full now that I have made friends with the Doctor." Two months later the same *igqirha* returned, showing Fitzgerald a stick with nearly one hundred notches that signified the number of patients he had treated since he was last at the hospital.[39] The exchange of knowledge went both ways: Fitzgerald was convinced that "the native doctors possess a great experience and knowledge both as to the treatment of many diseases on the one hand and the medicinal properties of plants on the other."[40] Fitzgerald even hoped to become head of the Xhosa doctors.[41] At first the weak structures of colonial rule ensured that colonial medicine negotiated its passage through African healers. The *amagqirha* retained an African framework for the transmission of new therapeutic technologies.

Another early mediator between European and Xhosa medicine was the paid employee. Most important were the interpreters who provided an invaluable linguistic and cultural bridge between Fitzgerald and the Xhosa doctors and patients. A little more than a month after the visit of Maqoma (son of King Ngqika) and his wife and daughter, Fitzgerald employed his son,

Ned Maqoma, as an interpreter.[42] Xhosa doctors like Gota came to trust Fitzgerald because of the presence of Ned Maqoma.[43] Although Fitzgerald paid them "salaries," these "workers" maintained a degree of autonomy and local notables like Ned Maqoma probably viewed themselves more as emissaries than paid employees. Ned Maqoma allegedly told Fitzgerald that he was so appreciative of his work that he would "remain with you as long as you stop in this country."[44] After Ned Maqoma died, still in Fitzgerald's service, another interpreter, Lot Rhai, took his place. These interpreters were nurses and some learned to carry out minor surgical operations, especially dentistry. But most significantly, through their role as cultural intermediaries, these individuals defined the nature of contact between African and European medical cultures. Nineteenth-century European medicine was to a certain extent Africanized

To be sure, colonial medicine retained its European core. For the 35 years that he ran the colonial hospital, Fitzgerald never relinquished his Victorian vision of establishing a well-ordered hospital that would heal while spreading "civilization." In 1859 he completed the permanent hospital where Africans arrived as in-patients to heal their most serious ailments. Fitzgerald's Victorian sense of order, combined with his miasmatic theories of atmospheric pollution as the source of disease, informed how the hospital was built and run. Large wards and ceilings that sloped towards an opening over which a ventilator was placed were required, for flat ceilings, according to Fitzgerald, were "pernicious in practice" as foul air cannot escape and "passes down and mixes up again with the pure air of the room, rendering it impure and unfit for the recovery of health."[45] So important was a pleasant smelling environment that Fitzgerald eventually had permanent canvas marquees constructed in which bad-smelling patients could be accommodated so as not to infect other patients.[46] He also developed a sewerage disposal system to separate solids and fluids and prevent cesspools which "fermented" and thereby released noxious vapors.[47] While the miasmatic theory behind much of this activity went against the rising dominance of germ theory in Western medicine, it did have the important effect of ensuring a hygienic environment conducive to healing, especially after surgical operations.

Fitzgerald was also convinced that the hospital needed to be a pleasant and comfortable area for recuperation (hardly surprising since Fitzgerald and his daughter lived in the South End of the hospital and Dr Egan, the District Surgeon, occupied the North End in exchange for services rendered).[48] He created a homely environment by adorning the walls with landscape paintings and placing flower pots all around the hospital to lighten the "dull heavy appearance of bare walls," with something "elevating and cheerful to look on ... [which] contributes much towards the recovery of their health."[49] On the arrival of patients Fitzgerald insisted on the provision of clean blankets and, when the finances were secured, proper hospital clothing.[50] Select patients were even supplied with screens to ensure privacy.[51] Nurses, initially African men, but then women trained by a European nurse, Mrs Ellen Parson, cared for the patients.[52] This strange white hospital, with its paintings of the English countryside, clearly conformed to the doctor's idea of a suitable place to practice and live and must have been strange to patients accustomed to smoke-filled thatch houses. Nevertheless, unlike the leper colonies, it never cut ties between the patients and their communities; visitors and patients were always free to come and go. For Africans, the hospital easily became a comfortable place to recuperate from illness or injury.

The most common disease of in-patients was syphilis followed by enteric complaints and a variety of skin conditions indicative of dietary problems possibly linked to protein deficiency.[53] Nearly half of all deaths in the hospital were due to respiratory ailments, probably tuberculosis.[54] The most serious epidemics were the occassional outbreaks of smallpox, which, for at least two hundred years prior to the colonization of south-eastern Africa, had swept across the area with much-debated consequences.[55] Given the famines of the 1850s, smallpox could have been particularly lethal if not for the intervention of Fitzgerald who, by the middle of 1858, had embarked on a widespread vaccination program.[56]

The hospital was relatively successful in helping to cure the patients admitted. The overall mortality rate was an average of 6.4 percent for African patients and 5.7 percent for European settlers with surprisingly low case fatality rates for a variety of diseases.[57] Probably the most efficacious treatment that the hospital offered was a well-balanced diet. At the hospital, every day patients received a substantial portion of potatoes, meat, vegetables, bread, barley, and milk. While initially rations were given to patients who, if able, prepared the food themselves or had family prepare it for them, the administering of food gradually became rationalized and cooks were employed. Fitzgerald had long recognized the importance of nutrition in aiding recovery and one of his enduring struggles with the Colonial Office was to ensure continued finances for the meals of the non-paying, African patients.[58]

In later years when finances were squeezed, Fitzgerald began to concentrate the provision of medical services to Africans at the dispensary (one possible explanation for the slightly higher mortality rate for African hospital patients is that only more serious African cases would be admitted into the hospital). Not only was the dispensary more cost-effective, but many African patients did not want to remain in the hospital for long periods of time.[59] As in the hospital, respiratory complaints were common, although for famine years a high number of enteric cases could be expected. A number of patients came for minor dental and aural complaints, ophthalmic problems, tapeworm, and skin problems. Fitzgerald and his aids supplied medication that relieved the symptoms of colds and respiratory complaints and carried out minor surgical operations from the removal of teeth to tumors. Between 1856 and 1884 the dispensary provided basic relief to the everyday ailments of over 85,000 Africans. From our admittedly unreliable census figures, an estimate of the African population two days walk from the hospital (a radius of 30 miles) suggests that from 70 to 90 percent of all Africans in this area were treated for some ailment (although evidence does show some came from farther away).[60] With the most meager resources, and in the face of an increasingly antagonistic state, Fitzgerald, in his peculiar fashion, had succeeded in establishing a public health care service.

Xhosa patients and doctors had, in a pragmatic fashion, chosen which therapies were effective and incorporated these into their everyday medical experience, on both a physical and cultural level. The new hospital dealt with these complaints with varying degrees of efficacy, which ultimately determined whether the Xhosa would continue to use the services provided. The structures of the medical collaboration forged in the 1850s continued to allow successful healing into the 1880s and beyond. The Xhosa recognized the advantages of Western medical care.

The rise of the settler colonial order

The entire story is not so sanguine; as early as 1853 the roots of the historical forces that would conspire against a fruitful exchange between African and European medical cultures can be identified. The advance of colonial settler forces and the creation of a "progressive" European medical system entwined in a new apparatus of power transformed the fortunes of this peculiar European–African medical encounter.

Among the Xhosa the firsts sign of resistance to and disenchantment with European medical services occurred during the Cattle-Killing prophecies. According to the believers of the prophecies, there was no need for colonial medicine, for health would be restored to all once the ancestors rose from the dead.[61] The number of people who visited the dispensary more than halved as the prophecies of Nongqawuse spread.[62] And, although the numbers that came to the dispensary increased after the First Disappointment in August 1856 when the ancestors failed to come forth, they declined again towards 1857 as faith in the reincarnation spread once again (Figure 3.1).

Only after the Second Great Disappointment in February 1857 did starving, emaciated Xhosa patients return to the hospital. The famine following the Cattle-Killings was so devastating that to one observer it seemed "that the prophecies had indeed come true, that the dead had risen from their graves at last, and were walking towards King William's Town."[63] They came to the hospital to seek relief from famine and starvation, not for the vague promises of Fitzgerald's mild remedies. The famine marked Fitzgerald's first great disappointment in his medical mission. For those who came to the dispensary, Fitzgerald could do no more than administer his standard treatment for the horrific symptoms of famine: a tablespoon of burnt brandy and hot ginger tea.[64] George Grey, intent on sending the Xhosa to work in the Cape, prevented Fitzgerald and other settlers in King William's Town from establishing a relief committee.[65] As Fitzgerald watched the

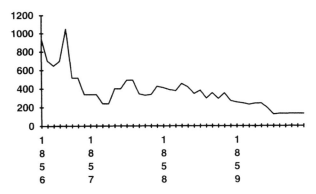

Figure 3.1 Number of monthly dispensary cases from 1856 to 1859.

Sources: CA CCP 1/2/1/18 A16–67 Hospital Reports, 1857–9; HGK 6/2, King William's Town Dispensary Book.*

Note
* 1856 begins in May. Figures for August 1856 from BKM, Fitzgerald's Letter Book, Fitzgerald to Maclean, 30 Aug. 1856; September from Fitzgerald to Maclean, 30 Sept. 1856; October and November total is 1,033 which is averaged at 516 from Fitzgerald to Maclean, 6 Dec. 1856. Dec., Jan. and Feb. 1857 average of balance of 1,011 patients. Averages also for 1857, March and April (477); May and June (795); July and August (982).

Xhosa die of starvation while the colonial government refused to administer aid and prevented private charity, his benevolent vision of curing the African sick must have been dealt a severe blow. He wrote to Chief Commissioner Maclean:

> The dead bodies I have seen lying about on the hill sides. . . . The scenes of misery and distress which I have witnessed, the cases I have been called upon to attend, the dysenteric and putrid atmosphere we have lived and breathed for the last few months, the truck loads of dead bodies almost daily being wheeled away to the burial ground cannot easily be effaced from one's memory.[66]

After the recent Great Potato Famine in his native Ireland (1846–51), the epidemiological consequences of the Xhosaland famine were no doubt clear to Fitzgerald.[67] Perhaps Fitzgerald also began to realize the limitations of his medical mission in the face of the social costs of the colonization and proleterianization of the Xhosa. Healing, of any sort, could play only the most limited ameliorating role when confronted by the greater forces of conquest, colonization, and the coming of capitalism, which underlay the changing patterns of morbidity and mortality.

The Cattle-Killing episode damaged Xhosa faith in colonial medicine and began to transform the nature of European–African medical collaboration in King William's Town. Xhosa doctors lost their trust in colonial medicine and Fitzgerald was less able to transmit technology within the existing framework of African medicine. Nevertheless, Fitzgerald continued to insist on the value of African medicine and as late as 1860 campaigned for the legalization and professionalization of African doctors who could be instructed in European therapeutic practices. Moreover, he contended that European medicine should not be forced on Africans and that the colonial authorities should "remove all prohibitions from the native practitioners" – a curious stance given George Grey's initial intention of reducing the authority of the *amagqirha*.[68]

When faced by continued colonial opposition to the legalization of African medical practitioners, Fitzgerald attempted to provide European medical training to select Africans who could then become both healers and bearers of the new civilization. He chose two missionary-educated youths – one was the son of Gota the *igqirha* – for formal training in England, but failed to secure sufficient funding from the colonial government.[69] However, the colonial administration showed less interest in what they began to perceive as an expensive "civilizing" project that paid few political dividends. Many in the Colonial Office felt that a hospital for Africans did not deserve the luxuries of the King William's Town Hospital and attempted to reduce the allocated expenditure. The problem was exacerbated by a change in alignment of colonial politics. Grey, beset with a personal scandal, ended his term as Governor of the Cape in 1861 and his zeal for the "civilizing mission" was not as ardently shared by the next Governor, Wodehouse. Grey's collaborators like Colonel Maclean lost their influence after the Cape annexed British Kaffraria in 1865. Moreover, the discovery of diamonds began to drag the attention of the Cape government from the eastern frontier to the northern hinterlands. Fitzgerald lost his old patrons in the colonial state and his role in the machinations of colonial rule seemed less justified. The result was a reduction in the government grant which forced the hospital to cut back on staff and begin to admit more paying European patients – by 1867 the number of African patients had dropped below that of Europeans. Although the Xhosa retained an interest in European therapies, resources for their treatment were being reduced (Figure 3.2).

Even while his appeals appeared increasingly anachronistic, Fitzgerald continued to promote Grey's civilizing schemes, for he thought that only the promises to eradicate witchcraft and "civilize" the "Natives" could "justify it [the hospital] for the large expenditure it [the government] incurs in connection with this department."[70] He persisted in attempting to train African doctors; every other year he pleaded with the Cape government for funds. A few Cape liberals remained sympathetic to his cause. However, when the Cape liberals finally agreed in 1877 to provide funds for the training of African doctors, the Ninth Frontier War between the colonialists and the Ngqika and Gcaleka Xhosa broke out. The plan was delayed and a disappointed Fitzgerald bowed to settler prejudice. In 1877 he wrote the Supreme Medical Committee that "I have no doubt myself of their intelligence and ability, and, if properly trained and educated, I should be

54   David Gordon

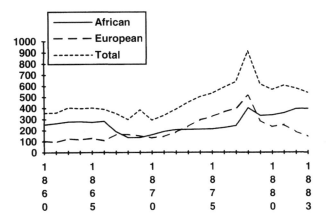

Figure 3.2 Number of African and European in-door hospital cases, 1860 to 1883.
Source: CCP 1/2/1/20–48, Hospital Reports, 1860–83.

Note
Number of Europeans exceeds Africans first in 1867, hovers around equal numbers, and only definitively falls below again after 1878. The rise in cases in 1878 is due to the Frontier War. Numbers of European patients then dropped below African as the colonial authorities made other medical services available to Europeans.

disappointed if the young men did not distinguish themselves in the study of the medical profession."[71] In 1878, following the outbreak of war, he conceded to settler prejudices and wrote that "it would be extremely difficult to find young men of sufficient advancement in civilized life and of sufficient education for the highest branches of the profession."[72] By the 1880s the broader colonial context had put an end to further negotiation between colonial medicine and African healers. The plan to train an independent corps of African doctors lay in ruins and the delivery of first-rate medical services at the Eastern Cape was increasingly restricted to European settlers.

Even though the King William's Town Hospital presents us with a moment in the history of medicine in the colonial territories that points to a possible alternative outcome to the accepted route of colonial medicine, in the longer term there was little possibility of a successful collaboration between medical cultures. As settler power grew and the colonial state solidified, European doctors eschewed African medical culture and African patients were offered second-rate care. The death-blow to the peculiar frontier hospital was delivered in 1891 when, after 35 years of service in Xhosaland, Fitzgerald retired and returned to England where he died in 1897.[73] Dr Ben Baine arrived fresh from the diamond fields of Kimberly to take charge of the hospital. Baine immediately modernized the hospital: he segregated wards for European and African patients, replaced African nurses with Europeans, and allotted smaller food rations to African patients.[74]

Conclusions

The early years of the King William's Town Hospital show how colonial medicine could become part of the therapeutic world of the Xhosa without destroying their cultural identities and spreading colonial hegemony. This chapter has outlined the rise of therapeutic choice during early colonization; how, in the words of Shula Marks, "African healers and patients were adept at adopting and adapting those aspects of Western medicine that worked without allowing this to undermine belief in the efficacy of their remedies and belief system."[75] In spite of the intentions of its promoters, colonial medicine in nineteenth-century Xhosaland was not an effective instrument of colonial hegemony. Rather, at first, it provided new surgical techniques, some pharmaceutical agents, and a few good meals. African healers and sufferers accepted the humanitarian offer of early colonial medicine without succumbing to its web of political intrigues.

In the late nineteenth century, Western medicine became rooted in the germ theory that Fitzgerald had always disdained. A "progressive" science supported by a growing settler colonialism emerged out of the new mining industries and came to taboo what had previously been useful so that it could carve out its own distinct "modern" identity. A discourse of modernity marked its boundaries by representing a "savagery" ossified in tradition. The medical culture of the European conquerors became soldered to the ideological machinery of that typical colonialism which would, over the next century, define South Africa's "development" against the backdrop of a native "backwardness." But, as many historians of South Africa have previously pointed out, that is a story of the twentieth century.

Notes

1 South African Library, Cape Town (henceforth SAL), MSB 223 B(10), Grey Collection, 21–2, Fitzgerald's manuscript "The Witchdoctors of South Africa"; Fitzgerald, *A Short History of the Native Hospital and Permanent Canvas Marquees* (King William's Town, 1885), 16; *King William's Town Gazette*, 10 Jan. 1857, 3.
2 Fitzgerald listed most of his African patients as "Xhosa," followed by "Fingo" (Mfengu). These ethnic distinctions do not faithfully translate social realities in the nineteenth century. Yet it is useful to distinguish Xhosa from Mfengu. In 1853 the Xhosa had only just been conquered and the colonial authority in Xhosaland was tenuous; by contrast, the Mfengu collaborated more closely with the colonial regime. For a history of Xhosa/Mfengu relations see Les Switzer, *Power and Resistance in an African Society: The Ciskei Xhosa and the Making of South Africa* (Madison, WI: Univesity of Wisconsin Press, 1993).
3 See Figure 1 (p. 52) for total numbers during the first 3 years.
4 British Kaffraria Museum, King William's Town (henceforth BKM), Fitzgerald's Letter Book, Fitzgerald to Grey, 7 May 1856. Most of these letters are also contained in Cape Archives, Cape Town (henceforth CA) BK100/1.
5 In 1888 the hospital was named the Grey Hospital after its most important sponsor. Here I retain the name King William's Town Hospital. The following article does not attempt to be a history of the hospital but an analysis of the

political forces, ideologies, and cultural prectices in which it was immersed. Those interested in a general history should consult BKM Box W6940, A. W. Burton, "A Brief History of the Grey Hospital," and Fitzgerald, *A Short History of the Native Hospital and Permanent Canvas Marquees* (King William's Town, 1885).
6 Jeff Peires, *The Dead Will Arise: Nongqawuse and the Great Xhosa Cattle-Killing Movement of 1856–7* (Johannesburg: Ravan Press, 1989), 60.
7 Influenced by Michel Foucault, such scholars view the development of European medical institutions as being integral to the construction of colonial power. For example, see Timothy Mitchell, *Colonising Egypt* (Berkeley, CA: University of California Press, 1991). For cases that deal specifically with medicine in the colonies, see David Arnold, *Colonizing the Body: State Medicine and Epidemic Disease in Nineteenth-Century India* (Berkeley, CA: University of California Press, 1993); and Megan Vaughan, *Curing their Ills: African Power and Colonial Illness* (Cambridge: Cambridge Universitry Press, 1991).
8 Arnold, *Colonizing the Body*, 292–3.
9 John M. Janzen, *The Quest for Therapy in Lower Zaire* (Berkeley, CA: University of California Press, 1978). On the relationship between "modern" and "traditional" medicine also see Murray Last and G. L. Chavanduka, *The Professionalisation of African Medicine* (Manchester: Manchester University Press, 1986).
10 For the relationships between the Xhosa and the land and labor requirements of settler farmers and miners see Colin Bundy, *The Rise and Fall of the South African Peasantry* (Berkeley, CA: University Of California Press, 1979); and Clifton Crais, *The Making of the Colonial Order: White Supremacy and Black Resistance in the Eastern Cape, 1770–1865* (Cambridge: Cambridge University Press, 1992).
11 The rise of therapeautic certainty in Western medicine and its cultural impact is best described in Edmund D. Pellagrino, "The Socio-cultural Impact of Twentieth-Century Therapeutics," in Charles Roseburg and Morris Vogel, eds, *The Therapeutic Revolution: Essays in the Social History of American Medicine* (Philadelphia, PA: University of Pennsylvania Press, 1979), 245–66.
12 Fitzgerald's manuscript remains unpublished in the Grey Collection of the South African Library, SAL, MSB 223 B(10), Fitgerald's manuscript, 29–64.
13 The seminal anthropological work is Victor W. Turner, *The Drums of Affliction: A Study of Religious Process Among the Ndembu of Zambia* (Oxford: Oxford University Press, 1968). John M. Janzen has three important books: *The Quest for Therapy in Lower Zaire* (Berkeley, CA: University of California Press, 1978); *Lemba 1650–1930: A Drum of Affliction in Africa and the New World* (New York: Garland, 1982); and *Ngoma: Discourses of Healing in Central and Southern Africa* (Berkeley, CA: University of California Press, 1992). A valuable work in the Nguni (Zulu) context is Harriet Ngubane, *Body and Mind in Zulu Medicine: An Ethnology of Health and Disease in Nyuswa-Zulu Thought and Practice* (London, 1977). In the Nguni (Pondo) context, Monica Hunter, *Reaction to Conquest*, 2nd edn (Oxford: University Press, 1961). A valuable section on healing among the Nguni (Xhosa) is in J. H. Soga, *The Ama-Xosa: Life and Customs* (Lovedale: Lovedale Press, 1931), 145–82.
14 Janzen identifies this collective feature of Ngoma as "therapy group management." Janzen, *The Quest for Therapy*, 51, 73.
15 The use of this particular chant has remained a central feature of Nguni medicine. It was recorded by Fitzgerald in the 1850s, by Soga in the 1920s, Monica Hunter in the 1930s (as *Siya vuma. Phosa ngemva*, we agree, put it behind), Harriet Ngubane among the Zulu in 1970s (she recorded *Ngiyavuma* which has the subject "I" instead of "we"), and Janzen in the 1980s. SAL,

16 SAL, MSB 223 B(10), Fitzgerald's manuscript, 29–64. There was some overlap; for example, a refusal to obey a calling would invoke ancestral wrath. Patients with a calling could also be "eaten" by the river-spirit (a form of possession). My account has been enriched by the anthropological works listed in note 15 and by Monica Hunter's work on the nearby Pondo, *Reaction to Conquest*, 320–48, 496–502.

17 Jeff Peires claims that cases were rare between 1853 and 1856, *The Dead Will Arise*, 62. In 1846 Kona, son of Chief Maqoma, allegedly burnt and strangled to death a senior counselor. He later told the story to Fitzgerald. Fitzgerald's manuscript, 1–6. In 1859 four men were found guilty by the Criminal Court of British Kaffraria of torturing a women to death by tying her up and lighting a fire under her arms and legs after accusing her of bewitching a child. These cases were collected by Grey to justify expenditure on the new hospital. SAL, MSB 223 B(9), Copy of the Proceedings of the Criminal Court of British Kaffraria, King William's Town, 12 April 1859. Also see Soga, *The Ama-Xosa*, 180–1.

18 For example see Fitzgerald, *A Short History of the Native Hospital*, 4.

19 SAL, Fitzgerald's manuscript, 30, 38, 51, 54, 56, 61; Soga, *The Ama-Xosa*, 160, 171; Hunter, *Reaction to Conquest*, 337–9.

20 Janzen also identifies the "phased rite of passage," which includes a number of stages as the central feature of Ngoma. He comments on the ability of Ngoma to adapt or employ treatments of different efficacy, *Ngoma*, 85–107, 153–72.

21 For a discussion of these issues and a cautionary note regarding the tendency of anthropologists to reduce African medicine to the equivalent of biomedicine see Robert Pool, "On the Creation and Dissolution of Ethnomedical Systems in the Medical Ethnography of Africa," *Africa* 64(1) (1994): 1–20.

22 Quoted in Robert Donaldson, "Dr John Patrick Fitzgerald: Pioneer Colonial Doctor, 1840–1860," MA thesis, University of Waikato, 1988, 23.

23 R. J. Towers, "Dr John Patrick Fitzgerald," *New Zealand Hospital*, Sept. 1964: 7–10; Robert Donaldson, "Dr John Patrick Fitzgerald," 1–138.

24 This is implied in some of the letters Fitzgerald sent to George Grey. Fitzgerald had a deep affection for Grey who cared for him after the death of his wife. In these letters Fitzgerald also implies that the Cattle-Killing episode may have been an outcome of Grey's attack on the *amagqirha* or a deliberate plot by Grey. While I remain skeptical, this does seem to provide the strongest evidence behind the "Grey's plot" theory of the Cattle Killings popular among Xhosa. See SAL, Grey Collection, 2(61), Fitzgerald to Grey, 16 July 1885, 10 April 1886, 19 July 1891, 30 Jan. 1893, 24 Dec. 1895. For an account of the "Grey's plot" theory, see Peires, *The Dead Will Arise*, x.

25 BKM, Fitzgerald's Letter Book, Fitzgerald to Maclean, 20 April 1856; Fitzgerald to Grey, 7 June 1856. For later reflection on this relationship see SAL, Grey Collection, 2(61), Fitzgerald to Grey, 16 July 1885, 10 April 1886, 19 July 1891, 4 Dec. 1895.

26 BKM, Fitzgerald's Letter Book, Fitzgerald to Maclean, 13 April 1856.

27 SAL, Grey Collection 6(61), "Letter from a Kaffir to the Queen," 14 July 1856.

28 Peires, *The Dead Will Arise*, 71.

29 Ibid., 78–209.

30 CA, HGK 6/2, King William's Town Dispensary Book.

31 Fitzgerald, *The King William's Town Hospital Reports: No. 1* (King William's Town, 1858), 10; *King William's Town Gazette*, 10 Jan. 1857, 3; BKM, Fitzgerald's Letter Book, Fitzgerald to Maclean, 19 May 1856; Fitzgerald to Maclean, 1 Feb. 1861.

58   David Gordon

32 Arnold Fischer, E. Weiss, S. Tshabe, E. Mdala, *English–Xhosa Dictionary* (Cape Town, 1985); J. McLaren, *A New Concise Xhosa–English Dictionary* (Cape Town, 1963 [first 1915]). A comparison with Zulu, the closest language to Xhosa, is instructive. Zulu medicine also employs the *vuma* chant which also means consent. However, there is no special name for opthalmia, and the noun *imvuma* is listed by Colenso as the animal slaughtered when a marriage is agreed upon. J. W. Colenso, *Zulu–English Dictionary* (Natal, 1905), 649.
33 J. McLaren, *A New Concise Xhosa–English Dictionary*; C. M. Doke, D. M. Malcolm, J. M. A. Sikakana, and B. W. Vilakazi, *Zulu–English Dictionary* (Johannesburg, 1990).
34 Robin Horton, "African Conversion," *Africa* 41 (1971): 57–108.
35 Franz Fanon, *Studies in a Dying Colonialism* (New York: Grove, 1989), 45.
36 Accounts of the meetings were written by Fitzgerald and were self-congratulatory. Nevertheless, it is unlikely that they were fabrications. *King William's Town Gazette*, 10 Jan. 1857, 3.
37 SAL, MSB 223 B(10), Fitzgerald's Manuscript, 23.
38 BKM, Fitzgerald's Letter Book, Fitzgerald to Maclean, 27 May 1856.
39 SAL, MSB 223 B(10), Fitzgerald's Manuscript, 23–6.
40 *King William's Town Gazette*, 10 Jan. 1857, 3.
41 BKM, Fitzgerald's Letter Book, Fitzgerald to Maclean, 2 March 1857.
42 BKM, Fitzgerald's Letter Book, Fitzgerald to Maclean, 20 April 1856; Fitzgerald to Grey, 7 June 1856.
43 Gota dreamt that Maqoma was to be found residing with Fitzgerald. SAL, MSB 223 B(10), Fitzgerald's manuscript, 21. Fitzgerald recognized that "Ned Macoma's knowledge of the Natives and influence combined with his avid zeal and interest in the success of the hospital materially aid me in my work." Unfortunately for Fitzgerald, Ned Maqoma died four years later in 1860. BKM, Fitzgerald's Letter Book, Fitzgerald to Maclean, 13 Jan. 1860; Fitzgerald to Maclean, 15 Aug. 1860.
44 Fitzgerald, *A Short History of the Native Hospital*, 16.
45 CA, CCP 1/2/1/21 G-9–69, Hospital Reports.
46 Fitzgerald, *A Short History of the Native Hospital*, 8–9.
47 He called this the "dry earth system," see Fitzgerald, *Sanitation, or Scavenging Simplified: The Method Adopted at the Native Hospital, King William's Town, South Africa* (King William's Town, 1886), 1–30.
48 CA, CCP 1/2/1/21 G-9–69, Hospital Reports.
49 CA, CCP 1/2/1/45 G-3–81, Hospital Reports; BKM, Fitzgerald's Letter Book, Fitzgerald to Colonial Secretary, 18 Jan. 1881; Fitzgerald to Under Colonial Secretary, 21 Jan. 1884.
50 BKM, Fitzgerald's Letter Book, Fitzgerald to Maclean, 28 June 1860.
51 Ibid., 23 April 1860.
52 S. Marks, *Divided Sisterhood: Race, Class and Gender in the South African Nursing Profession* (London: Macmillan, 1994), 80.
53 Calculated from CA, HGK 6/2-3 Dispensary Book; CA, CCP 1/2/1/18 A16–67, Hospital Reports. For account of primary stage syphilis see Fitzgerald, *The King William's Town Hospital Reports*, 19. For both syphilis and respiratory complaints, African and settler infection and fatality seem to have been of a similar nature, although fatality for respiratory complaints among Africans was slightly higher than for the settlers and settlers suffered from more enteric complaints.
54 The respiratory complaints were roughly distributed between what Fitzgerald termed catarrh, pneumonia and pthisis. Together with the high case fatality rate – between 15 and 35 percent – and the reasonably close correspondence between African and European cases, the prevalence of virulent pulmonary tuberculosis seems likely. There was a total of 281 African respiratory cases compared to 210

A sword of empire? 59

European cases with average case fatality rates of 18.9 and 17.1 percent respectively. A sample of exclusively African dispensary patients' cases taken in 1858, 1864, and 1867 confirms that most Africans trekked to the hospital because of respiratory complaints. Calculated from data from CA, HGK 6/2-3 Dispensary Book; CA, CCP 1/2/1/18 A16–67 Hospital Reports.

55 The first detailed records of a smallpox epidemic are from the 1713 epidemic which supposedly decimated the Khoi. The effects of this epidemic are still being debated. Andrew Smith, "Khoikhoi Susceptibility to Virgin Soil Epidemics in the Eighteenth Century," *South African Medical Journal*, 75(1) (1989): 25–6. The spread of disease in the wake of famine may be due to both a tendency to migrate to find food, thus spreading disease or becoming susceptible to new diseases, and weakened resistance due to under nourishment. For study in the Southern African context see Elizabeth Eldredge, "Drought, Famine and Disease in Nineteenth-Century Lesotho," *African Economic History*, 16 (1987): 61–93.

56 He distributed vaccine to nearby missionaries and within King William's Town he supervised the vaccination of around 600 people every week. For the smallpox campaign, see G. S. Hofmeyr, "King William's Town and the Xhosa: The Role of a Frontier Capital," MA thesis, University of Cape Town, 1981: 128–32; Also *King William's Town Gazette*, 26/06/1858, 1/10/1858, 23/10/1858.

57 Mortality rates for all hospital cases between 1867 and 1877 calculated from CA, CCP 1/2/1/19 to 35. For comparative material on hospitals in England and the "hospital debate" surrounding their efficacy see S. Cherry, "The Hospitals and Population Growth: The Voluntary General Hospitals, Mortality and Local Populations in the English Provinces in the Eighteenth and Nineteenth Centuries," *Population Studies*, 34 (1980): 59–75, 251–65.

58 BKM, Fitzgerald's Letter Book, Fitzgerald to Grey, 7 June 1856; Also see Fitzgerald's address, "To all the Natives of Port Nicholson and other places" quoted in Towers, "Dr John Patrick Fitzgerald," 8; Cory Library, Fitzgerald, *Hospital Reports: No. 1*, 12; BKM, Fitzgerald's Letter Books, Egan to Fitzgerald, 15 Oct. 1863, Fitzgerald to Brownlee, 28 Oct. 1863; CA, HGK 3/10, Blaine to Colonial Office, 16 May 1892. The administrator, Dr Blaine, who replaced Fitzgerald in 1891 wanted to reduce these rations. CA, HGK 3/10, Blaine to Colonial Office, 16 May 1892.

59 Fitzgerald claimed that "The natives have all sorts of foolish prejudices and ungrounded fears about remaining in hospital," CA, BK 101, Fitzgerald to Brownlee, 19 May 1862.

60 This figure calculated from 1856 until 1884. The number supposedly reflects different patients as no repeated entries in the dispensary book were made. CA, CCP 1/2/1/19 to 55; BKM, Fitzgerald's Letter Book, 21 Jan 1884, 13 Jan. 1885. For the entire period of Fitzgerald's administration up until 1891, Fitzgerald claims he treated over 130,000 cases. This is not unlikely as the number of patients visiting the dispensary in the 1880s was increasing. SAL, Grey Collection 2(61), Fitzgerald to Grey, 19/07/91. Jeff Peires, following Theal, claims the Xhosa population declined from 105,000 to 38,500 in the famine following the Cattle-Killing. A colonial census of 1875 puts the non-white population in 1,781 square miles around King William's Town at 97,628. Peires, *The Dead Will Arise*, 328; Theal, *History of South Africa*, Vol. 3, 206; CA, CCP 1/2/1/30, Hospital Reports.

61 SAL, Grey Collection, MSB 223, B(10), Hospital Anecdotes, n.p.

62 See Figure 1 (p. 52). In July 1856, there was a marked decline in the number of Xhosa patients who were usually the majority of Fitzgerald's patients. The number of "Khoi" and "Mfengu" patients who did not believe in the Cattle-Killing continued to rise. Also see BKM, Fitzgerald's Letter Book, Fitzgerald to Maclean, 6 Dec. 1856.

63 Peires, *The Dead Will Arise*, 245.
64 BKM, Fitzgerald's Letter Book, Fitzgerald to Grey, 7 July 1856. For specific treatments of these patients see CA, HGK 6/2, King William's Town Dispensary Book.
65 Peires, *The Dead Will Arise*, 241–72.
66 BKM, Fitzgerald's Letter Book, Fitzgerald to Maclean, 15 Sept. 1857.
67 Ibid., 28 Feb. 1857.
68 BKM, Fitzgerald's Letter Book, Fitzgerald to Fielding, 4 April 1860.
69 Fitzgerald, *The King William's Town Hospital* (1864), 5–8; BKM, Fitzgerald's Letter Book, Fitzgerald to Colonial Secretary, 31 Aug. 1868.
70 CA, BK 101, Fitzgerald to Egan and Peters, 11 Sept. 1860.
71 CA, CCP 1/2/1/33 G-64–77, Hospital Reports, 1877.
72 CA, CCP 1/2/1/55 G-15–83, Hospital Reports, 1878.
73 *Cape Argus Weekly*, 13 Jan. 1897.
74 CA, HGK 2/4 Blaine to Colonial Office, 3 March 1892. Catherine Burns argues that the 1928 Medical, Dental and Pharmacy Bill finally solidified state control over the right to heal and undermined the legitimacy of more informal healers. Catherine Burns, "Louisa Mvemve: A Woman's Advice to the Public on the Cure of Various Diseases," *Kronos*, 23 (1996): 108–34, 121.
75 Marks, *Divided Sisterhood*, 80.

4 Midwives, missions and reform
Colonizing Dutch childbirth services at home and abroad *ca.* 1900

Hilary Marland

The guiding theme of this chapter is that it is not necessary to go far afield to discover a 'colonial' situation or a 'mission' to reform. This is not a particularly novel notion. It has been shaped and analyzed in different contexts, with 'colonization' and the imposition of administrative structures at home and abroad being seen as important building blocks in the construction of the modern state. In a recent article summarizing work on medicine in colonial settings, Shula Marks asked the pertinent question 'What is colonial about colonial medicine?'.[1] For Roy MacLeod and Milton Lewis, medicine is 'an instrument of empire', 'an imperializing cultural force' and colonial medicine is about 'the experience of European medicine overseas'.[2] David Arnold adopts a different stance, placing indigenous experience and the role of agency centre stage, and suggesting that the barrier between colonial and metropolitan medicine is by no means rigid. Rather, what was happening in the colonies – in Arnold's case, India – mirrored the ideological and administrative processes that went into the building of modern states, particularly Britain.[3]

'Colonial' endeavours are ubiquitous in nineteenth and early twentieth-century European states. Philanthropy can be seen as a mission into the darker reaches of society, the imposition of Christianity, cleanliness and bourgeois ethos on an irreligious, grubby and unruly rabble.[4] Bible, nursing, visiting and missionary societies were set up to cleanse the urban slums, 'where disease and irreligion were rife'.[5] Educating the urban poor meant efforts towards redemption through teaching, the victory of learning over ignorance, instructing the unkempt and ignorant – the 'residuum', 'street arabs' and the 'dangerous and perishing classes' – to take their orderly place in urbanizing society.[6] The 'them' and 'us', the lurking 'other' permeates the development of nineteenth-century towns, the division of urban space, fear of crime and the spread of disease.[7] It was a divide which was enormous and threatening, yet at the same time one which contemporaries saw as being vital to bridge. In medical practice too, the re-invention of the medical profession in the mid decades of the nineteenth century also set the scene for a campaign to guide away the misguided masses from the lure of quackery toward modern, rational, scientific and hygienic medicine.[8]

Comparing the reform of midwifery in a 'home' and 'overseas' context offers a means of exploring the idea that not only charity, but also missionary enterprise begins at home. Observing the reform of midwifery in the context of the poor southern provinces of the Netherlands and the Dutch East Indies,[9] chiefly the island of Java, enables us to compare and contrast what were in effect parallel efforts, which commenced and gained momentum at the turn of the twentieth century. In this chapter, perceptions of the problems, the need for and language of reform, and (albeit sketchily) proposed solutions will be explored. Due to the strictures of chapter writing and accessibility of data (much work remains to be done on almost all aspects of Dutch colonial medicine), analysis of reform in both contexts will be through the lens of the reformers only, in their efforts to improve maternity care by bolstering the supply and quality of midwives.

In 1897 the Dutch set about the task of reforming Dutch maternity services in their East Indies colonies in response to concerns about the high levels of both infant and maternal mortality. At the same time, they redoubled their efforts to improve the standard of midwifery care at home. In both contexts, reform turned upon the agent of the midwife, herself to be reformed through teaching, before embarking upon her missionary work either at home in the poor predominantly Catholic regions to the south of the country or abroad. Like Bible-women, the midwives were to be 'native agents'[10] drawn largely from the districts where they would later return to practice. Through the process of becoming a professional midwife during a two year school training (three years after 1921), the identity of these young women as model and modern midwives would be forged and made explicit to the pupils themselves, their 'traditional' rivals, and the populations amongst whom they would work.

There is a striking overlap in the chronology of the Dutch 'midwife question' at home and abroad, particularly in the appearance of influential reports on midwife practice, status and future roles in both settings in 1897 and 1909–11. Each set of reformers showed an awareness of the efforts of their opposite numbers, which were widely reported in the medical and lay press. Elements of competition between those involved in the two reforming movements can be detected; the colonial reformers in particular stressed that they had homed in first on the need for reform and the manner of executing this reform. And in the essence of the reforms – perceived problems and solutions – useful analogies can be drawn. The language of reform is 'virtually' interchangeable. Yet a direct criss-crossing of information and ideas, and the anticipated links between reformers in the two contexts have proved elusive. The separateness of the services, the sense of difference which captured the mood of medical reform in the colonies, and the complexity of providing coverage in the East Indies, overrode the potential for cooperation; and besides colonial solutions were often more imaginative and diverse, and predated Dutch attempts to reform midwifery services.

The urge to reform midwifery services at home in the deprived southern provinces of the Netherlands, Limburg and North Brabant, gained momentum in the late nineteenth century.[11] Reform took on new meanings in the south, where improving midwifery services was a raw struggle, which overrode the issues of competition between doctors and midwives, of defining tasks, maintaining national standards, or even following legislation. The means of solving the problem of defective maternity services was simple – to supply trained midwives in sufficient numbers – but it was to prove enormously difficult to implement. The need for midwives in the south led local reformers to diverge from national policy-making to seek their own solutions. Their language became one of missionary endeavour, of seeking to supply a basic service to the local population, an endeavour strongly tinged with the perceived necessity of recruiting local ('native') girls, of transforming them through training, and placing them back into the setting from whence they came to reform their own people. The mission in the southern provinces was a Catholic enterprise, bent not just on improving conditions for childbearing women, but also on ensuring the survival and blossoming of 'Catholic motherhood' in the region.[12] The word 'colony' can be skewed and applied to the south, not to describe a political fact, but a feeling of separation; not a geographical distance, but a perception of distance.

The difficulties of supplying midwives to the countryside, particularly in the south, had been acknowledged in reforming national legislation during the nineteenth century. The Health Acts of 1818 and 1865, and the act setting up the first state school in Amsterdam in 1861, reiterated the need to train girls up and get them out to the areas where they were most needed,[13] but setting up of the state schools for midwives in Amsterdam and Rotterdam did not produce results in the south where there remained a critical shortage of midwives. Those who had work in the south, laboured on the land for little return, or in the mines and cotton factories of Limburg, and trained midwives were not keen to work in areas dominated by unemployment or under-employment, need and poor housing. For the midwife, this meant bad working conditions and low financial returns. One doctor writing from Amsterdam in 1909 remarked that in the south 'most [read: all] parishes were too small or too poor to support a midwife'. How, he asked, could midwives be persuaded into a position where they would 'starve from hunger' in the needy parishes of Limburg?[14]

The southern provinces were depicted in striking terms. The border began with the 'great rivers' of the Maas and the Waal. There was an other-worldliness to the south: predominantly Catholic compared with the Protestant north, poor in the extreme and, according to contemporary reports, often those of doctors writing on the health practices of the region, 'primitive', 'dangerous' and 'superstitious'. The impact of poverty and traditionalism on health was striking and has been well-documented by Van Poppel and other Dutch historians and demographers.[15] Infant mortality was almost double that of the more prosperous western provinces of the country.[16] Great variation between villages within the province were attributed by observers to the impact of quacks and the old women who interfered in birth and infant care.[17] They also pointed to problems of deficient education, alcohol abuse, the employment of women in factories and the negative influence of Catholicism:[18] the breast-binding of young girls, exposing sickly children unnecessarily to ensure a quick baptism, and the feeble response of Catholics to sickness and disease compared with the businesslike health-promoting actions of the Protestants.[19] A recent study of the Brabantine Kempen describes the claustrophobic sense of shame which developed during the second half of the nineteenth century amongst Catholics, the obsessional repression and shrouding of the female body, which made it impossible for women to breast-feed.[20] Within – yet also apart from – the Netherlands, the southern provinces of North Brabant and Limburg were, as regards health care, a colony at home.

The problems of the south were a source of great embarrassment locally and nationally, but they were interpreted in very different ways by local reformers as compared with the distant central government and health administration. The pleas of local men for support and their struggle for reform resemble in many ways those of colonial administrators: they felt distanced, different, separate, neglected, excluded. With respect to maternity services, Dr Clemens Meuleman, who would become the first director of the midwife school in Heerlen, commented that, compared with three centuries of midwife training in the north and west, the south had nothing. No training, few midwives, few doctors and great poverty and need. The only thing the south had more of was deaths.[21] The campaign for a school in the south dated from late in the nineteenth century,[22] and raised much opposition as national interests were weighed up against local concerns. Various initiatives to set up schools in Limburg and North Brabant were resolutely blocked. Expectations were lower in the south, which stung both government and the national midwives' society, who were keen to uphold standards. Dr Woltering, chief health inspector for the southern provinces, argued in a blunt minority note to the government's advisory panel on health, the *Gezondheidsraad*, that overall standards would possibly be lowered by initiatives in the south, but that the level of obstetric care in the region would be improved. This, for Woltering, was the key issue.[23]

In 1913 a school was finally established in Heerlen in Limburg, close to the major town of Maastricht, under the auspices of the *Vereeniging Kweekschool voor Vroedvrouwen* (Society to establish a training school for midwives). The region was at the core of the Catholic reform movement, and the midwife initiative was firmly supported by the committee of the Jozef's-hospitaal, also based in Heerlen. Though the founding of the Heerlen school was urged by the Catholic minister of the interior, Jhr. Ch. Ruys de Beerenbrouck, and partially funded by the state and a provincial subsidy, its existence depended chiefly on an enormous private and Church input. Medical director Meuleman, a vigorous Catholic and force for the reform of all aspects of maternity care, had a vital role in setting up the school. He was president of the committee for *Sociale Kinderhygiëne*, active in all aspects of infant welfare, and the founder of a refuge for unmarried mothers which was linked to the school; above all he was depicted, especially by the Catholic press, as a 'friend of all children'.[24] Convinced of the hopelessness of relying on government support, Meuleman saw state subsidies as playing only a supplementary role in his 'mission' to reform the south. The school came to be organized with the express purpose of promoting Catholic motherhood, encouraging Catholic births, ensuring attendance by Catholic midwives, resisting birth control and enabling baptism, while at the same time urging modern hygienic standards intended to save mothers and babies.[25] The problems anticipated by opponents of a school in the south did not go away: it was difficult to achieve appropriate standards amongst the pupils, and problems of distribution and competition were sometimes exacerbated rather than improved. Midwives trained in Heerlen simply failed to go where they were supposed to, preferring the more prosperous districts in the west of the country where practice returns were better.[26]

The Heerlen school was defined in terms that we can liken to a mission. Without the enormous input of the Catholic Church and Meuleman's 'pressing urgency' it is unlikely that a school would have opened in the south during this period. He described how 'the three midwife schools above the rivers'[27] were attended by few pupils from the south and they also supplied few Catholic midwives'.[28] In 1910 more than a third of women gave birth in Limburg and North Brabant without midwifery help.[29] In Limburg the situation was described by Meuleman as 'pitiful', with only 58 midwives for a population of over 300,000, and neither a doctor nor midwife in 123 out of 176 parishes.[30] It was crucial to have women of the same faith provide attendance in childbed. The extra number of midwives required to fulfil the 'mission' was closely calculated by the Church authorities – in 1925 to a total of 335 – as leading figures in the Catholic Church allied themselves closely to the school directors in promoting Catholic motherhood and guiding the work of Catholic midwives.[31] A Catholic midwife would be trained to carry out emergency baptisms and to support the Catholic mother: in the words of Meuleman's successor, Dr C. J. Lubbers, 'a midwife who is sincere and deep in her Catholic belief, has a powerful influence on her environment'.[32] Local churchman provided more spiritual and invigorating explanations of the mission. In 1934 the Heer van Haaren, a local chaplain, addressing the Catholic Midwives Society, the 'congregation of Mary's children', urged midwives to 'Save them, the needy, through your love, not through words, not through pleas and speeches; though Christian motherhood and love the woman will be saved'.[33]

There are striking parallels between the writings of reformers on the need for initiatives in the Dutch colonies and those encouraging improvements in the south of the Netherlands. There is a good deal of literature on both reform movements to inform us.[34] For the Dutch East Indies, Verdoorn's lengthy thesis of 1941, *Midwifery help for the native population of the Dutch Indies*, is especially useful.[35] In the south and in the colonies the late nineteenth century was marked by stepped up interest in the 'midwife question', triggered by concern over high infant mortality rates and the loss of mothers' lives; the trained midwife was seen as the solution in both contexts. The commencement of the debate in the Netherlands is usually dated as 1897, with the production of a report by the Dutch Society for the Promotion of Medicine,[36] which analysed the position of midwives and sought ways of improving this through raising levels of practice, fees and status. Less well known is the fact that this was preceded by a similar report and lively debate on midwifery practice in the Dutch East Indies.[37] Already by the late nineteenth century many varied methods of tackling the problem of supplying midwives had been tried out in the Indies.

The debate in the Dutch East Indies led to a reiteration of a range of ideas on how to develop midwife training, quite different from the monotonal solution reached in the Netherlands, based solely, after 1861, on admission to midwife schools and the abandonment of apprenticeship or training in other institutions. Some colonial doctors, including H. B. van Buuren, author of the 1897–8 reports, firmly advocated training schools, and the school solution dated back to the establishment of a dedicated institution for midwife training in the capital, Batavia, in 1850. Admitting around twenty local girls each year, the training (as in the Netherlands after 1861) was to be for two years, with an emphasis (as at home) on teaching the basics of reading, writing and arithmetic in the first year, combined with theoretical midwifery and practical experience. The hope was that the girls once qualified and working in their districts would make 'Western midwifery' so popular that more pupils would be sent to the capital for training. The results, however, were modest: by 1873 a total of 142 young women had been admitted to the school, but only half of these remained in practise. Most worked in the more populous districts of Java, so their distribution was limited, but nearly all were said to function well. Still, not enough were being recruited and in 1875 the school was abandoned as being too expensive, despite pleas to reactivate the programme, based on offering midwives guaranteed salaries and supporting them through the distribution of propaganda.

Some ten years later, in 1886, the question of training indigenous women was raised once again, this time based on the idea of private teaching by 'European' doctors, who would be remunerated for each pupil taken on. Instituted in 1891, by 1897, when the 'midwife question' resurfaced, fourteen midwives had been trained under this scheme. In the Netherlands, where, by the close of the century, small numbers of pupils passed through school training each year – no more than 60 to 70[38] – improvements in supply were discernible in much of the country. But in the Indies, the impact of such small numbers of trained midwives carrying out an average of only twenty-four deliveries a year went virtually unnoticed. Yet hope was expressed that the scheme could be expanded quite easily; and in 1897 when the 'midwife question' became prominent once more, the debate largely centred around the relative merits of private versus school training.[39]

In 1897 the *Algemene Handelsblad*, one of Holland's leading daily newspapers, raised the issue of standards of maternity care in the colonies, under such titles as 'White and brown *Indische* mothers' and 'The mothers in Indië'. It was reported that

> European and native women in our East Indies possessions pass far too often into the hands of the unqualified at deliveries; most midwives do not even fulfil the most basic requirements ... Delivered up to ignorance and coarseness, to fanaticism and superstition, suffering and death amongst women, literally speaking, is the order of the day.[40]

These, in the words of Verdoorn, 'unexpected' articles, brought the issue of the training of indigenous midwives in the Indies to the attention of the Dutch public, and set off a chain reaction. The issue once raised in the Netherlands, resulted in swift and diverse responses in the Indies, producing a large body of literature, including two substantial reports by Dr H. B. van Buuren, on the 'midwifery question' in the Dutch Indies.[41] In concrete terms it led to the extension of provision for the training of local girls as midwives by European doctors.[42] In 1910 there were 97 working midwives in the Indies, a number which rose to 697 by 1938, or at an average rate of 21 a year.[43] Training followed a variety of routes. Some women trained first as nurses, before following an extra course in a hospital, clinic or nursing mission; others followed a school training, or were trained privately by a doctor or qualified midwife.

A variety of options for training remained built into the East Indies solution. It could hardly be otherwise in such a diverse, scattered, widespread colony, much of it untouched and unknown, where medical help was provided by the government of the Indies, supplemented by local initiatives, and the work of missionary societies and the Red Cross.[44] As an alternative to Indies-based solutions, Dr Monnikendam in a speech delivered at the national exhibition on women's work held in Amsterdam in 1898, specifically opposed the setting up of a school in the Indies, mooting instead the idea of training midwives in Holland for work in the colonies. A small number of Dutch midwives, trained in the Netherlands, worked in the mission overseas, mostly in religious orders, but this remained an insubstantial group.

Others believed that maternity care could best be organized by Dutch women doctors trained in obstetrics, whose brief would be to train indigenous girls to deliver babies.[45] By 1925 there were thirty-five women doctors working in the Dutch East Indies, including the influential N. Stokvis-Cohen Stuart, who settled in Semarang, Java in 1908. Shocked by the terrible state of obstetric care and nursing for infants, she raised money in the Netherlands to set up a training school for indigenous nurses and midwives. A brilliant propagandist, who enlisted the help of Islamic activists, the prominent Djokjakarta dynasty and the Dutch Red Cross, she established clinics, not just for pregnant women and infants, but for poor patients in general, created the Society for the Improvement of Native Nursing and wrote a textbook for use by her trainees. The type of work Stokvis-Cohen Stuart carried out was recommended as being highly suitable for Dutch women doctors, an appropriate channel for female practise; 'the native wishes in the first instance for a woman's help for his wife and children'.[46]

A number of commentators picked up on the fact that the 'midwife question' was raised first and responded to most vigorously in the Indies rather than the Netherlands, and it was also pointed out that while the colonial situation was dire, obstetric services at home were far from rosy; 'Was it not the general complaint in Europe, that the standard of midwives was still at a very low level!'[47] Striking too is the language of reformers in both contexts as they describe the problems of providing obstetric care and the solutions offered. Within or outside the schools, the key was to train 'native' girls, young malleable women who were easily moulded into childbirth missionaries, yet who would be working amongst their own kind to reform childbirth and rid the local population of traditional practices and traditional attendants.

Doctors seeking reform in both contexts spoke of the 'bad', 'dangerous' and 'superstitious' practices surrounding childbirth. These were typically doctors moving into a 'colonial' situation, either from more prosperous districts of the Netherlands with more thoroughly developed obstetric services, or from the Netherlands overseas. In 1927 one general practitioner, H. R. Folmer, reflected back on his experiences thirty years previously, when 'as an inexperienced doctor' he came from Amsterdam, fresh from his medical training, to the 'then still primitive region and people' of Zuid Beveland in Zeeland. He reflected the curiosity, disbelief and despair which confronted doctors witnessing traditional 'folk' practices for the first time.[48] Most pregnant women in Folmer's district reached full-term without being examined by a doctor or midwife, women gave birth on the ground, and if a doctor could not attend an 'old woman' would step in; 'assistance then consisted largely of pulling and stretching the soft parts' by a tippling or cigar-smoking midwife.[49] Describing common practices in Limburg surrounding pregnancy, birth and lying-in, Starmans remarked on the frequency of popular beliefs, tinged with superstitious practices, the influence of time, weather and heavenly constellations on the birth, mixes of prayers, medicine and rituals to ensure good outcomes.[50] P. A. Barentsen, writing in 1935, simply described the population of Kempenland in Brabant as 'less developed people', and spent the next 366 pages explaining why.[51] In essence, these doctors were describing a 'colonial' situation, and their words echo those of colonial doctors witnessing similar conditions from a 'western' perspective.

Writings on midwife practice in the Dutch Indies have a similar tone. Van Buuren remarked on how the deeper inland one went the worse the attendants were. Expectant approaches were rare, and he was shocked by the rough practices of the 'native' midwives, who were described as old crones, dirty, diseased and ignorant. To illustrate this, Van Buuren included photographs of thirty traditional midwives, *doekoens*, practising in the division of Kediri in his report. Most obviously, these women were severely malnourished and elderly; Van Buuren pointed out that most were over 50, and some much older.[52] Of the total of 278 *doekoens* in Kediri, many were blind or syphilitic, several were crippled or paralysed on one side; some had lost their noses as a result of disease: 'They were a sorrowful group to see'.[53] In 1937 a report on maternity care in Dessa, regretted that 'the mentality of the population is little changed over the past 30 years: stupidity, superstition, clinging to tradition, conservatism and fear are normally the reason why when help is first called for it is very late or too late'.[54]

The identity of the modern trained midwife in both contexts was to be quite different from her traditional counterpart. The *dorps vroedvrouw*, village midwife, and her dreadful accomplice, the *baker*, the unqualified dry nurse, of the southern provinces of the Netherlands, had more than their equals in the *doekoens* of the Dutch East Indies. These women were depicted as the greatest barriers to reform, but also as being unconscionably popular amongst the women they assisted. They represented a tie with traditional ways which needed to be broken. 'The natives in general would rather have the hocus-pocus of the *doekoens*, most old sticks', who 'butchered' their patients, than midwives trained in European ways. The village midwives were trusted as, 'older women, who had themselves had children'.[55] The solution to the evils of the aged crone, and her misinformed, rough and superstitious practice, was the young midwife, transformed and trained up in modern ideas of hygiene and practice. The attributes which age could bring of experience, maturity and knowledge were dismissed by reformers, as part of a wider shift from the early nineteenth century onwards (in connection with midwife and nurse training) away from emphasis on the value of maturity and experience acquired by older women who had themselves borne children, to the model of easily influenced and teachable young women, blank pages to be written on.[56] Age limits were imposed in the Netherlands and the Dutch East Indies for admission to training programmes. At the Heerlen school, candidates were admitted between the ages of 19 and 26; in the Indies, girls as young as 16 were taken as pupils. And results were quickly claimed for the success of training programmes involving young 'native' women. After just 1 year of training, Van Buuren was claiming good results for two midwives, who had been instructed to keep accounts of their cases. Djasminah and Tasminten recorded with pride their use of hygienic and 'Western' methods. Tasminten, who could not write, must have dictated her case reports:

> The Chinese woman Goudee called me at 9.00 in the morning. The delivery of the child and placenta carried out by a *doekoen*. The woman is dizzy, short of breath, the pulse is very faint and quick. While I rubbed the uterus, the people on my instruction showed me the placenta, from which a large piece was missing. Therefore I carried out a quick

disinfection of my hands, went with my right hand in the uterus, peeled loose a large piece of remaining placenta, which was solely responsible for the bleeding.[57]

These women, and many other midwives, related their efforts to measure the pulse carefully, to disinfect and irrigate with lysol, to insert catheters, to administer chloroform; they also remarked disapprovingly on the work of the *doekoens*, and on the fact that the women they delivered were often syphilitic and clung to superstitious practices.

Training could take much longer in the Indies, which was one reason reformers emphasised the advantages of starting young; by the time she was 21 a young woman could be fully trained.[58] Her responsibilities, as Stokvis-Cohen Stuart was quick to point out, could be considerable; the midwife had to take more on, because there was simply no choice. Isolated from doctor colleagues, and without encouragement to reinvigorate her studies through journals and refresher courses, lacking a textbook in her own language, she still had to continue to practise efficiently, and carry out difficult procedures, including the application of forceps and repair of perineal tears.[59] These procedures were denied to Dutch midwives by law, though many carried them out, arguing that they had no choice when they were working in isolation without access to medical assistance.[60]

Commentators were keen to banish the misconception that either the tough rural population of the southern Netherlands or the indigenous population of the Indies had an easy time in childbirth. 'Let me immediately release you from this dream', remarked Stokvis-Cohen Stuart.[61] Like European women, Indies women sometimes had narrow pelvises, but luckily their children were also on the whole smaller; otherwise a colleague remarked, 'the misery would be impossible to overview'. But they suffered regularly due to malpresentations, long deliveries, placenta praevia, and most often from the attentions of the *doekoens*.[62] Mortality figures were sufficient to show the fallacy of the idea of 'native' women having problem-free births. Data on death rates amongst birthing women are very difficult to interpret and figures vary enormously, but there was agreement that mortality was likely to be much higher in isolated areas. In 1935 one estimate claimed that 37 per cent of indigenous women delivered with qualified attendants, but these deliveries would be concentrated in the towns and more populous areas.[63]

A survey published in 1933 divided mothers into two groups: those who had been examined during pregnancy, and those who had not, the later group including undetected complications of pregnancy and difficult deliveries, and the majority of unfavourable presentations. Overall the maternal mortality rate was 71.3 per 10,000, 295 per 10,000 for the group who had not been examined previously.[64] Professor R. Remmelts recorded an overall maternal death rate of 90 per 10,000 in the Indies, taken from cases reported by a number of midwifery services between 1931–5; these rates compared with 20–30 per 10,000 in the Netherlands between 1923–7.[65] The southern provinces of the Netherlands had the worst maternal mortality (and infant mortality) rates, of the country; in Limburg between 1917–26 the rate for the province was 27 per 10,000 compared to the national rate of 25, but rates varied enormously from village to village as they did in the Indies, and this was blamed chiefly on the interference of traditional attendants.[66]

A file on the 'midwife question' has been preserved in the archives of the Dutch National Bureau for Female Labour. Between the years 1906–17 the file chiefly contains newspaper cuttings reporting on 'Obstetric help in the south' and the 'New midwives school' juxtaposed alongside 'The midwifery question in the Dutch Indies'. Clearly the compilers of this scrap book saw a link between the movements to reform midwifery at home and abroad; it was a link which could hardly be overlooked.[67] Standards of colonial midwifery and the midwife question in the Netherlands were revived together at a meeting in Leeuwarden in 1909,[68] which led to extensive discussion of midwifery in the Dutch Indies in the same year, and to a report on the status of the midwife in the Netherlands in 1911,[69] coinciding too with the fruition of plans for the Heerlen school. Analogies are limited largely to describing the essence of the problems and solutions; there is scant evidence of direct interaction or exchanges. A few individuals crossed between the two parallel trajectories, notably Professor Hector Treub, one of Holland's most distinguished obstetricians and a staunch supporter of the reformed midwife, who worked for change at home and abroad. Closely involved with the Heerlen initiative (and Clemens Meuleman's thesis supervisor and thus mentor), Treub was also an enthusiastic advocate of the school solution in the East Indies.

In the 1930s the Heerlen school, having concentrated on and learned the missionary enterprise at home, extended its work to the colonies. Dutch girls trained at the school went out to the colonies, and from 1934 young women were sent from Curaçao to Heerlen and returned there following three years of training. Three years later the first pupils were sent from the Dutch East Indies to the school. The numbers trained in Heerlen who took up colonial work, however, remained small; by 1955 a total of only 16 had been sent to Indonesia, 11 to the Dutch Antilles (9 of these to Curaçao), 1 to Suriname and 2 to South Africa.[70] Emphasis was placed on the need to send not just Dutch midwives, but Catholic midwives to the colonies. The Catholic midwife could work well in different 'missionary fields', which 'did not always require the same tasks and working environment'. And 'the more civilized natives seem already to prefer a Roman Catholic midwife'.[71]

Parallel responses to the problems of colonial midwifery encountered parallel difficulties. The geographical and cultural differences between the two settings were striking, yet reformers talked in both contexts of the hard task of getting midwives to the areas where their work was needed, and of steering them away from more prosperous 'developed' towns. The training process itself raised expectations, in terms of living standards and midwives' perceptions of their future status as local health professionals. The notion of bringing in local girls, training them, reforming them and sending them back as childbirth missionaries contained much potential for conflict. Competition for custom between general practitioners and midwives was less at issue in either context, as many districts lacked either a midwife or a doctor, and doctors were often heavily involved in the campaign to get midwives into their areas. Yet school-trained midwives were brought into direct conflict with the traditional childbirth practitioners, who were by no means easily got rid of. And in both contexts the difficulties of keeping the trained midwives true to what they had learnt were enormous once they returned to their own villages or districts. While some midwives had difficulties putting into practice what they had learnt, others were simply not accepted in the areas where they worked. Stokvis-Cohen Stuart remarked upon the problems of young 'emancipated' women being accepted, particularly when they moved to new areas after training, especially the islands other than Java, with their different populations, different religions, other languages, other customs.[72] Midwives writing letters back to the school directors in Heerlen grumbled of similar barriers to acceptance at home: problems in finding a place to practise, partly because of resistance to a Catholic midwife f there were not enough Catholic mothers in a district, or because their methods did not fit, a fondness for the old traditions, or because of attachment to the old midwife and her way of doing things.

Incomes could be poor in both settings, and midwives had a struggle to build viable practices. In the East Indies midwives were generally paid a fixed sum by the government for their work, plus a fee for each case; in 1905 it was recommended that the 'native' midwives' income be raised from 10 to 15 guilders a month, plus 2.50 guilders for each 'native' delivery and 5 for attending the birth of a European woman.[73] The free market, or a combination of a town post with private practice, was usual at home. Many midwives working in the south found it hard to make ends meet, and town councils, knowing the limits of private practice, offered large salaries, way in excess of larger towns in the west of the country, as incentives.[74]

Ex-pupils wrote regularly to the Heerlen school directors from their missions at home and abroad, describing their practice and financial experiences. Sister Susanna, who qualified from the Heerlen school in 1941, was described during training as 'poor in examinations and below average, but cheerful and handy'. She expressed her intense disappointment at not being sent to a colonial posting. In a poignant set of letters, she traces her career as a district nurse, work she had done before training as a midwife, making the best of her training by encouraging the mothers she visited to breast-feed, but always worried that she would loose her midwifery skills. Her contemporary Sister Cecilia wrote each Christmas of her hopes of being sent on a mission overseas, but remained at a general hospital in Drenthe.[75] Other midwives reached the colonies via a circuitous route. Theresia van Krieken, who also qualified in 1941, worked first in Helmond, grumbling at the lack of work there, subsequently hunted for other posts, but by 1944 was expressing her pleasure in her work and growing caseload. She sold her practice in 1947, needing the money to enter a convent, and in 1951 wrote as Sister Theresita, working in Hakassar in the local maternity hospital and the antenatal clinic in St Fatimah: 'it was', she declared 'wonderful work'.[76]

The mission at home could be tough and many of the girls working in the southern provinces had a long struggle to build up a viable practice and to establish themselves, yet there are success stories too. Nor should we imagine that midwives in the colonies always failed to prosper. There is little material in the Heerlen school archive on pupils' experiences in the East Indies, but there is an interesting file on the small number of women who travelled from Curaçao and Aruba to Heerlen, and after three years returned home to practice. O. Gonzalez, wrote in July 1937 of her work first in Aruba and then Curaçao. She remarked that it was easy to get her predominantly poor clients into hospital in emergencies, on the need for an infant welfare bureau, and that 'the population here is very wilful; sometimes you must resolutely stand up against old customs'. As well as her government salary, she had a private practice, and had just purchased a Chevrolet sedan from a retiring midwife.[77]

The 'missionary midwives' sent to reform 'indigenous practices' commanded considerable support. So great was the need for their services, that other considerations, their threat to the practices of local doctors, or the danger that they would overstep their brief and carry out medical tasks or attempt to deal with more complicated midwifery cases, were often overlooked as irrelevant to the main problem of supply. Indeed it was stated that the midwife in the Dutch Indies would require an even better training than her Dutch counterpart as once in practice in isolated areas she would be hard-pressed to find a doctor in emergencies: 'she would have to save what there was to save'.[78] Yet training, and follow-up, must have varied enormously. The problem of calling in a doctor in time and of midwives going beyond their competence in emergencies was remarked upon in isolated areas of the Netherlands too; by and large, a blind eye was turned to what was seen as a necessary evil.

Is it possible or reasonable to compare two areas which vary so much in scale, geography, history, culture and economy? After all, the southern provinces of North Brabant and Limburg were still part of the Netherlands, and part of an emerging Europe. They were poor and backward, but welfare provisions were being introduced, schooling extended. They were predominantly Catholic, while the rest of the country was by and large Protestant, but culturally they shared much with the rest of the country. Can we really compare this to the Indies, with its several hundred populated islands (although by and large this chapter is concerned with Java), its mix of populations, religions, and languages, its huge geographical spread and the inaccessibility of much of the archipelago? Yet the language used to describe the problems of introducing midwifery care to combat maternal and infant deaths coincide, and it is these ways of perceiving the problem and its solutions which have largely concerned me here. In both contexts the midwife was recreated in a new image as a modern reformed practitioner, a mediator entrusted with the task of reform, not just of midwifery practice, but also hygiene, infant care and general health standards, on behalf of the colonial administration or central government. This could be a flawed image, as midwives were depicted as potentially falling prey to traditional ideas when once again they were working back in the areas from whence they came. The historical texts speak in terms of difference in both contexts, of isolation, the problems of tradition and superstition are formulated and reformulated in the same way. We could argue as in Arnold's India where the imposition of modern medicine as a 'colonial science' took place in 'an exceptionally raw and accentuated form',[79] that conditions were accentuated in the Indies, higher up on the scale of dreadfulness, and the difficulties of reform much greater. One source writing in 1939 described how

> the task of the midwife here in the countryside is very different ... The people deliver in the most filthy environment, the darkest and smallest corner of the house, preferably on the ground (sometimes earth), in a sitting position and the native helper (a kind of midwife without any understanding) looks on hopelessly if the child or the woman dies.

This quote could come from either context, albeit one would expect it less in the south of the Netherlands as late as 1939; the language is interchangeable, the problems the same.[80]

Acknowledgements

This chapter was first presented at the Society for the Social History of Medicine 'Medicine and the Colonies' Conference, Oxford, July 1996. My thanks to Harriet Deacon and Molly Sutphen, and to the audience for their comments, and to the Wellcome Trust for their generous support of my project on Dutch midwives 1897–1941.

Notes

1 S. Marks, 'What is colonial about colonial medicine? And what has happened to imperialism and health?', *Social History of Medicine*, 10 (1997), 205–19, esp. 206–7.
2 R. MacLeod and M. Lewis (eds), *Disease, Medicine and Empire* (London and New York: Routledge, 1988), p. x.
3 D. Arnold, *Imperial Medicine and Indigenous Societies* (Manchester: Manchester University Press, 1988), and ibid., *Colonizing the Body. State Medicine and Epidemic Disease in Nineteenth-Century India* (Berkeley, Los Angeles and London: University of California Press, 1993), p. 9.
4 E.g. David Owen, *English Philanthropy, 1660–1960* (Cambridge, MA: Harvard

University Press, 1964); Frank Prochaska, *Women and Philanthropy in Nineteenth-Century England* (Oxford: Clarendon, 1980).
5 F. Prochaska, *The Voluntary Impulse. Philanthropy in Modern Britain* (London and Boston: Faber & Faber, 1988), p. 48.
6 J. Hurt, *Elementary Schooling and the Working Classes 1860–1918* (London: Routledge & Kegan Paul, 1979), p. 4.
7 See e.g. G. Stedman-Jones, *Outcast London. A Study in the Relationship between Classes in Victorian Society* (Oxford: Oxford University Press, 1971), and M. Poovey, *Making a Social Body. British Cultural Formation, 1830–1864* (Chicago and London: University of Chicago Press, 1995).
8 W. F. Bynum, *Science and the Practice of Medicine in the Nineteenth Century* (Cambridge: Cambridge University Press, 1994).
9 I have tended to use Dutch East Indies throughout, although the islands of the archipelago were first named Indonesia in modern times by a German geographer in 1884.
10 Prochaska, *Women and Philanthropy*, p. 126.
11 Some aspects are developed more extensively in my essay, 'The midwife as health missionary: between traditional and modern practices in early twentieth-century Dutch childbirth', in H. Marland and A. M. Rafferty (eds), *Midwives, Society and Childbirth: Debates and Controversies in the Modern Period* (London and New York: Routledge, 1997), pp. 153–79.
12 Hilary Marland, '"Catholic girls, there is work!": Dutch midwives, childbirth reform and Catholicism in the early twentieth century', unpublished paper, Plenary Talk, Conference 'Nursing, Women's History and Politics of Welfare', University of Nottingham, 18–21 September 1996.
13 M. J. van Lieburg and H. Marland, 'Midwife regulation, education, and practice in the Netherlands during the nineteenth century', *Medical History*, 33 (1989), 296–317.
14 J. G. I. Blaisse, 'Een nieuwe kweekschool voor vroedvrouwen', *Telegraaf*, 4 Dec. 1909.
15 F. van Poppel, 'Religion and health: Catholicism and regional mortality differences in nineteenth-century Netherlands', *Social History of Medicine*, 5 (1992), 229–53; R. Philips, *Gezondheidszorg in Limburg. Groei en acceptatie van de gezondheidsvoorzieningen 1850–1940* (Assen: Van Gorcum, 1980).
16 North Brabant is often cited as the blackest of the obstetric blackspots: M. Pruijt, 'Van vroedvrouw tot verloskundige. De ontwikkelingen in het vroedvrouwenberoep in Nederland in de periode 1865–1940', doctoraal scriptie, Katholieke Hogeschool Tilburg, 1987; ibid., 'Roeien, baren en in de arbeid zijn. Vroedvrouwen in Noord-Brabant, 1880–1960', in M. Grever and A. van der Veen (eds), *Bij ons Moeder en ons Jet. Brabantse vrouwen in de 19de en 20ste Eeuw* ('s-Hertogenbosch: Walburg, 1989), pp. 122–42; M. Pruijt, 'De verloskundige zorg in Noord-Brabant 1900–1940', *Sociale Wetenschappen*, 31 (1988), 175–93. In the years 1901–5 the infant mortality rate in North Brabant at 183 per 1,000 live births was the highest in the country, comparing with a national rate of 136 and 92 in the more urbanized and prosperous province of South Holland: C. Vandenbroeke, F. van Poppel and A. M. van der Woude, 'De zuigelingen en kindersterfte in België en Nederland in seculair perspectief', *Tijdschrift voor Geschiedenis*, 94 (1981), 481.
17 P. A. Barentsen, 'Over de kindersterfte ten plattenlande van Oost-Noordbrabant', *Nederlandsch Tijdschrift voor Geneeskunde* (hereafter *NTvG*), 66:IIA (1922), 612.
18 Methorst presented infant mortality rates for the Netherlands for the period 1907–10 which showed that this was 100 per 1,000 live births for Catholics, 70 for Protestants and only 55 for Jews: H. W. Methorst, 'Geboorte-acheruitgang

en Zuigelingenbescherming', *NTvG*, 60 (1916), 1241–48. Even in the post-war period lesser, but still significant, discrepancies have been recorded: D. Hoogendoorn, *De Zuigelingensterfte in Nederland* (Assen: Van Gorcum, 1959).
19 P. J. M. Aalberse, 'Kindergeboorten en kindersterfte', VI and VII, *Katholieke Sociaal Weekblad*, 35 (1917), 353–6; 37, 373–7.
20 P. Meurkens, *Sociale verandering in het Oude Kempenland: Demografie economie en cultuur van een preindustriële samenleving*, proefschrift, Katholieke Universiteit Nijmegen, 1984.
21 J. Kuypers, 'Uit de Geschiedenis van de R. K. Vereeniging "Moederschapszorg" te Heerlen', Bij gelegendheid van het 25-jarig jubileum 1912–15 Oct. 1937, *Moederschapszorg*, 14 (1937), 151–4.
22 J. H. Starmans, *Verloskunde en kindersterfte in Limburg. Folklore: Geschiedenis: Heden* (Maastricht: Van Aelst, 1930), pp. 143–61.
23 Archief van de Afdeling Volksgezondheid en Armenwezen, 442. Nota, als bedoeld in art 14 van het Kon. Besluit van 27 Mei 1902, stll. no. 77, van het lid van den Centrale Gezondheidsraad, Dr P. M. J. M. E. Woltering. See H. Marland, 'Questions of competence: the midwife debate in the Netherlands in the early twentieth century', *Medical History*, 39 (1995), 317–37.
24 Notably in the special issue of *Moederschapszorg*, 9 (1932), following his premature death in the same year.
25 P. Boselie, 'Het ontstaan van de Vroedvrouwenschool te Heerlen', *Maasgouw*, 107 (1988), 142–58. For the characteristics of Catholic motherhood, see Marland, '"Catholic girls!"'.
26 See H. Marland, '"A broad and pleasing field of activity"? The payments, posts and practices of Dutch midwives in the early twentieth century', in J. Woodward and R. Jütte (eds), *Coping with Sickness. Historical Aspects of Health Care in a European Perspective* (Sheffield: European Association for the History of Medicine and Health, 1995), pp. 67–91.
27 State schools (*Rijkskweekscholen*) in Amsterdam (1861) and Rotterdam (1882). Groningen's school, attached to the university medical faculty, was established in 1851.
28 *Veertig Jaar R.K. Vereeniging Moederschapszorg. De Kweekschool voor Vroedvrouwen te Heerlen 1913–1955*, p. 18.
29 C. Meuleman, *De Kweekschool voor Vroedvrouwen te Heerlen en de kindersterfte in de Zuidelijke Provincien*, 1912.
30 Kweekschool voor Vroedvrouwen te Heerlen. 1e Jaarverslag, 1912–13, p. 9.
31 Archief Vroedvrouwenschool Heerlen (AVH), 52. Correspondentie met bisschoppen in Nederland. Nota omtrent het aantal R. K. Vroedvrouwen dat in Nederland benoodigd is, Nov., 1925.
32 'De vrouw en haar werkkring', *De Nieuwe Eeuw*, 8 March 1934.
33 'Waarom Kath. Vroedvrouwen Katholiek vereenigd?', *Maandblad voor R.K. Vroedvrouwen*, 11: 129, April 1934, 1136–42, pp. 1141, 1140.
34 Yet there is virtually no historical work on the 'midwife question' or many other questions concerning the provision of medical services in the Dutch colonies. One exception is G. M. van Heteren, A. de Knecht-van Eekelen and M. J. D. Poulissen (eds), *Dutch Medicine in the Malay Archipelago 1816–1942* (Amsterdam and Atlanta: Rodopi, 1989), which is largely concerned with the organization of services, medical teaching and specific diseases. Also still useful is D. Schoute, *De geneeskunde in Nederlandsch-Indië gedurende de 19de eeuw* (Batavia: Kolft, 1935).
35 J. A. Verdoorn, *Verloskundige Hulp voor de Inheemsche Bevolking van Nederlandsch-Indië: Een Sociaal-Medische Studie*, proefschrift, Rijksuniversiteit Leiden, 1941.
36 'Nederlandsche Maatschappij tot Bevordering der Geneeskunst. Rapport der

commissie ter onderzoek naar de wijze waarop door geneeskundigen, verbetering gebracht kan worden in het gehalte en positie der vroedvrouwen in Nederland', March 1987. In *NTvG*, 33:I (1897), 610–28.
37 H. B. van Buuren, *Het verloskundig vraagstuk voor Nederlandsch-Indië* (Amsterdam, 1897); ibid., *Nog iets over de verloskundige hulp in Nederlandsch Indië* (met een vooorrede van Prof. Hector Treub) (Leiden, 1898).
38 Van Lieburg and Marland, 'Midwife regulation', p. 307.
39 Verdoorn, *Verloskundige hulp*, pp. 97–111.
40 H. Bervoets, 'Verloskundge hulp ann Inlanders', *Geneeskundig Tijdschrift voor Nederlandsch-Indië*, 38 (1898), 357–8.
41 Van Buuren, *Het verloskundig vraagstuk*; ibid., *Nog iets over de verloskundige hulp*.
42 'Inlandsche vroedvrouwen', *Echo*, 8 June 1902.
43 Verdoorn, *Verloskundige hulp*, p. 213.
44 Before 1800 the VOC (Vereenidge Oost-Indische Compagnie, United East India Company), sent many surgeons and smaller numbers of doctors to the Indies. After 1816, and the short period of British rule (1811–16) during the Batavian Republic, former areas under the VOC in the Indonesian archipelago were ruled by the Netherlands Indies Government, directly answerable to the king and minister of the colonies in the Netherlands, and the VOC played virtually no part in the provision of medical services. See P. Boomgaard, 'Dutch medicine in Asia, 1600–1900', in D. Arnold (ed.), *Warm Climates and Western Medicine* (Amsterdam and Atlanta: Rodopi, 1996), pp. 42–64 for a broad account of the provision and reception of medical services in the Dutch colonies.
45 D. C. Nuysink-Steinbuch, 'De vrouwelijke artsen in Nederland en Nederlandsh Indië', *NTvG*, 70:IIB (1926), 2095–6.
46 Ibid., pp. 2095–6; N. Stokvis-Cohen Stuart, 'Vrouwelijke artsen voor Indië', *NTvG*, 74:I (1930), 1268–70.
47 Dr van Buuren, 'Een jaar verder', *Nederlandsh Tijdschrift voor Verloskunde en Gynaecologie*, 11 (1900), 1–46, p. 1.
48 H. R. Folmer, 'Volksgebruiken in Zeeland bij geboorte en kraambed', *NTvG*, 70:IB (1927), 3112–8.
49 Ibid., p. 3113.
50 Starmans, *Verloskunde en kindersterfte in Limburg*.
51 P. A. Barentsen, *Het oud Kempenland. Eene proeve van vergelijking van organisme en samenleving* (Groningen: P. Noordhoff, 1935).
52 Van Buuren, *Het verloskundig vraagstuk*.
53 'De doekens', *N. Rott. Courant*, October 1909.
54 'De verloskundige hulp in de Dessa in Nederlandsch Indië', *Geneeskundige Gids*, 15 (1937), 494–7, 496.
55 Verdoorn, *Verloskundige hulp*, p. 103.
56 See H. Marland, '"Stately and dignified, kindly and God-fearing": midwives, age and status in the Netherlands in the eighteenth century', in H. Marland and M. Pelling (eds), *The Task of Healing. Medicine, Religion and Gender in England and the Netherlands 1450–1800* (Rotterdam: Erasmus, 1996), 271–305.
57 Van Buuren, 'Een jaar verder', pp. 35–6.
58 N. Stokvis-Cohen Stuart, 'Vroedvrouw opleiding in Indië en verloskundig werk in Indische bevolking', *Tijdschrift voor Sociale Hygiëne*, 33 (1931), 76–94, 85.
59 Ibid., pp. 85–9.
60 See Marland, 'Questions of competence'; especially useful is a report of Professor Nijhoff, AVH, 13. Gezondheidsraad 1930–31. Commissie inzake bevoegdheid vroedvrouwen, No. 153/15. Betr. uitbreiding bevoegdheid vroedvrouwen, 26 May 1930.
61 Stokvis-Cohen Stuart, 'Vroedvrouw opleiding in Indië', p. 76.

62 'De verloskundige hulp in de Dessa', p. 495.
63 Ibid., p. 496
64 B. Walch-Sorgdrager, 'Eenige obstetrische gegevens over al of neit tijdens de zwangerschap onderzoche patienten van Boedi Kemoeliaän', *Geneeskundig Tijdschrift voor Nederlandsch-Indië*, 73 (1933), 1371–87, 1385–6.
65 R. Remmelts, 'Over verloskunde in Nederlandsch-Indië', *Geneeskundig Tijdschrift voor Nederlandsch-Indië*, feest bundel 1936, 146–55, 151.
66 Starmans, *Verloskunde en kindersterfte in Limburg*, pp. 256–78.
67 Internationaal Informatiecentrum en archief voor de vrouwenbeweging. Inventaris van de archieven van het Nationaal Bureau voor Vrouwenarbeid en de Nationale Vereniging voor Vrouwenarbeid: Vroedvrouwen, 764, 1230–1234, 1906–17.
68 *NTvG*, 8:II A (1911) (bijblad), 545–8.
69 'Rapport der commissie in zake het vroedvrouwenvraagstuk hier te lande, benoemd door het hoofdbestuur der Nederlandsche Maatschappij tot Bevordering der Geneeskunst in samenwerking met het bestuur der Nederlandsche Gynaecologische Vereeniging', February, 1911. In *NTvG*, 55:I (1911), 1105–32.
70 *Veertig Jaar R. K. Vereeniging Moederschapszorg.*
71 De missie-vroedvrouw', *Maandblad R. K. Vroedvrouwen*, 7:89 (Jan. 1930), 586–94, 594.
72 Stokvis-Cohen Stuart, 'Vroedvrouw opleiding', p. 80.
73 F. S. Stibbe, 'Verloskundige Praktijk in de Desa. Kritiek op het Rapport der Commissie tot Voorbereiding eener Reorganisatie van den Burgerlijken Geneeskundigen Dienst', *Geneeskundig Tijdschrift voor Nederlandsch-Indië*, XLIX (1909), 385–415, 393.
74 Marland, '"A broad and pleasing field of activity"?', esp. pp. 75–9.
75 AVH, 192. Geslaagde Vroedvrouwen, Cursus 1938–41: A. M. H. van Erven (alias Zr. Cecilia); Verschuren (alias Zr. Susanna).
76 AVH, 192. Geslaagde Vroedvrouwen, Cursus 1938–41: T. C. van Krieken.
77 AVH, Vroedvrouwen Curaçao; O. Gonzalez to Dr Lubbers, 21 July 1937.
78 'Het werk van een vroedvrouw op het platteland in Indië', *Tijdschrift voor Praktische Verloskunde*, 42:24 (1939), 470–2, 471.
79 Arnold, *Colonizing the Body*, p. 9.
80 I cheated, translating *doekoen* to native helper in this instance; 'Het werk van een vroedvrouwen op het platteland in Indië', p. 471.

5 New Zealand milk for 'building Britons'

Philippa Mein Smith

The imperial historian Sir Keith Hancock provided a spur for this research when he responded to my declared interest in cows and babies: 'what a wonderful subject for a young New Zealander'. Why did he, an Australian, think that?[1] The appearance of sculptured cows on the lawn beside the New Zealand High Commission in Canberra, Australia's federal capital, in the late 1980s reinforced the intuition that this statement was worth pursuit. Why cows? It transpired that the New Zealand High Commission bought the corrugated iron sculptures, by New Zealander Jeff Thomson, because of their popularity and talent for self-advertisement. According to the High Commission, 'they prompted a familiarity and a nostalgia about New Zealand'. Once 'grazing' on the back lawn of the Chancery in Canberra, the cows 'continued to draw comment and large crowds.'[2] These nostalgic responses, and even the few complaints that the cows damaged New Zealand's image in Australia, suggest that milk continues to be a symbol of identity for New Zealanders. Australians would not respond in the same way because of their divergent memories of childhood and 'home', and of a rural landscape internalised as dry and red rather than wet and green.

Historically Australia produced a different mix of staple agrarian commodities from New Zealand and so designed different advertisements to disclose its ideals.[3] As Avner Offer has outlined in his agrarian interpretation of the Great War, for Australia, as for Canada and Argentina, wheat was the 'great expanding staple of the Edwardian period'. 'New Zealand added meat and dairy products' to its primary exports.[4] More than Australia, it took up refrigeration and built dairy factories from the 1890s, which were etched on the countryside in landscape painting. Typical was Christopher Perkins' 'Taranaki' (1931), the white cone of Mt Taranaki with a dairy factory in the foreground.[5]

To understand how a small country like New Zealand formed its settler identity, it is necessary to see it within an imperial framework, as a supplier of food to Britain, the world's largest importer and global trader. Economically, the end of empire came much later in New Zealand than suggested by the markers of diplomatic history. New Zealand, a Crown Colony from 1840, became a British Dominion in 1907 and adopted the Statute of Westminster in 1947.[6] Britain obliged New Zealand to reconsider its position in the world rather late, in 1973, when it turned away from its empire towards Europe and joined the European Economic Community. A central point of this essay is that it is essential to consider political economy, unlike Foucault did, because a study of economic history illuminates power relations. As Ann Stoler demonstrates, Foucault's dismissal of political economy as a positivist relic circumscribed the power relations he saw at play.[7] A history of milk offers insights into how New Zealanders constructed their culture and identity.[8] From the turn of the century until the 1960s, New Zealand was the Empire's dairy farm.[9] Milk as a cultural icon became central to images of New Zealand as 'clean and green' and a healthy environment in which to bring up children.

This study explores ways in which the image of New Zealand milk – a product of settler capitalism in the temperate world[10] – articulated with national, racial, regional, gender and professional identities. It shows how medical arguments helped transform milk from an accessory and a luxury into an 'essential food'; an imperial icon of health for New Zealand and the British Empire; and a medicine to counter racial degeneracy. To consider milk as a food requires awareness of people's interaction with their environment, both physical, cultural and political. Claude Levi-Strauss stated that it was characteristic of humans 'to convert natural resources into cultural objects' and food is the first example of culture in nature.[11] Milk as a drink or a food was not the 'staff of life'; it could not be because it was not a carbohydrate. However, it had long possessed a 'mythic status' as a life-giving fluid, a food for invalids and especially for children that was pure and good.[12] This mythic association with health and purity was not surprising given the whiteness of breast milk and cow's milk and that, traditionally, mother's milk was essential for a baby to live and be healthy. In the twentieth century, when consumerism joined science and democracy as part of the modern world order,[13] milk became the food most symbolic of maternal and child welfare policies, of nourishment by the mother, the family and the state.

Significantly, New Zealand's emerging national identity centred on a reputation for social experiment. In the first half of the twentieth century this took the form of pre-eminence in maternal and child welfare. The interplay between this reputation in health and New Zealand's economic dependency upon the British market had the effect of transforming milk the commodity into an imperial icon of health and racial strength. Building the child and the nation, and a white world, were international concerns, which in New Zealand were inseparable from their imperial context.[14]

Milk was a food, a drink and a medicine, and above all a children's food. Metaphorically and practically in Western societies, milk was associated with mothering and nurture. Yet earlier this century dairy products were associated with health, strength and virility, when now the association is often with heart attacks and gallstones. This gendered paradox of milk's masculine and feminine virtues was reconciled by the contemporary significance attached to building better babies and strong bodies, bones and teeth in growing children, first for imperial prowess and national efficiency and, from the Second World War, for building a democratic world. At a time when the child was perceived as social capital, child welfare reformers, politicians and dairy farmers promoted milk as a nation and empire builder, as the food most likely to improve the nutritional status of future citizens. As late as 1955, the New Zealand Department of Health's first state nutritionist, Dr Muriel Bell, declared that milk was for 'building Britons'.[15] In a white Dominion which supplied food and soldiers for Britain, milk from the cow and the mother served as a medium between building children's bodies and the 'body politic'.[16]

Anthropologists recognise that our relations with food are 'one of the most common and pervasive sources of value in human experience';[17] and the effectiveness of a food as an ethnic symbol is a product among other things of the relationship between people and nature. Milk, as a food, can therefore be interpreted as a 'medium' that has helped express colonial and national identity.[18] New Zealand had the climate, grass and rainfall for dairy farming and put cows out in the sunlight and fresh air – like babies – an advertised difference from Europe. New Zealand's infant welfare authority, Dr Frederic Truby King, declared in 1905 that the 'broader principles of life apply equally to plants and animals', first testing his ideas about natural rearing on an audience of farmers to whom he appealed as the source of a 'strong, healthy, capable race', before mothers tried out his code.[19] His bevy of devotees subsequently provided patronage for his milk mixtures and clock-work rules for babies along the trade routes of the Empire.[20] In a colony that perceived itself as Britain's farm, professionals influenced by the eugenics movement readily made explicit the links between rearing young stock – animals – and children. Child health services, from infant welfare clinics to school inspections to health camps, were intent on 'fattening human stock' as public health shifted its focus from the environment to people, starting with babies and children, and their nutritional needs.[21] Milk was, and is, central to images of New Zealand as 'clean and green'. It is central to images of New Zealand as an agricultural producer and as a healthy place to bring up children, a healthy country which has realised the yeomen image, where people lead an active outdoors life.

Production as culture

Arguably it is in consumption rather than production where milk becomes cultural history, but my research has confirmed that these are inseparable. There is no question that production is a part of culture, in what it reveals about people and their environment, as work, and in shaping social and political life. In his study of sugar's change from a luxury to a necessity, Sidney Mintz found that production and consumption were so closely bound together that each partly determined the other.[22] For milk, as for sugar 100 years earlier, agro-industry in the colonies – this time, in the temperate rather than the tropical world – boosted certain capitalist classes in British centres of commerce.[23] The production of milk immediately raises the issue of colonialism, or 'ecological imperialism'.[24] Chopping down the bush to obtain pasture suitable for dairying and breaking in the land in the process of economic development entailed a colonial relationship with the land. Imperialising the landscape was relatively straightforward, for it was discovered that 'English grasses thrive wherever the natural bush and fern are cleared'.[25]

New Zealand promoted itself as 'The Empire's Dairy Farm'[26] particularly in the 1920s and 1930s because its meat and dairy products entered the world economy as products of empire, supplying British consumers 12,000 miles distant from the farms planted in English grasses which produced them; and because in its bilateral trading relationship with the Mother Country, New Zealand sent 79 per cent of its exports to Britain while 60 per cent of its imports were British in 1914.[27] In wartime, Britain commandeered all the surplus butter, cheese and dried milk that New Zealand could produce. When we consider where commodities were received, in peace and in war, dairy production was first and foremost for the British breakfast table and the mass end of the market, the working classes. New Zealand – forced to be a price-taker by its size – supplied half of Britain's cheese and a quarter of its butter in the 1920s.

The Dairy Export Control Board, established in 1923 to manage the marketing of dairy produce, made six 10-minute movies for Britain in the 1920s, including 'New Zealand: The Empire's Dairy Farm'. All six promoted the 'Fernleaf', a national brand which used a New Zealand emblem from the First World War when New Zealand soldiers were known as 'fernleaves', and all six films ended with a 'picturesque' sunset scene of an ocean steamer disappearing over the horizon, carrying produce to the United Kingdom.

> With the words, "Healthy stock – sunbathed pasture – rippling streams – assure ideal production," the first film plunge[d] into the portrayal of half a dozen beautiful herds. Magnificent purebred milking Shorthorns drop[ped] down a grasslined bank, and cross[ed] a running stream to spread fanwise over rich river flats, picturesquely dotted with clumps of native bush.[28]

The herds were large by European standards, demonstrating the success of agricultural development in the Dominion, and the films projected the settler conception of New Zealand as a 'land of natural abundance'.[29]

In a sense the movies showed how a British export, grasses to New Zealand, were re-imported decades later in another form, New Zealand milk. In between, grass and cows helped process an imperial identity. One film acknowledged this in its title, 'The Dairy Cow as an Empire Builder'. It opened with the supposedly 'romantic' line: 'Where Maori warriors fifty years ago held at bay English troops – to-day their descendants make a daily round gathering cream cans!' Explicitly stated was that 'Butter for Britain wrought the change' from 'former wilderness' to 'to-day's development'.[30] The 'Empire' represented what had been created in New Zealand by providing for the British table: civilisation of the wilderness and of the indigenous people, the Maori, were the outcomes of producing food for British needs.

The movies represented 'a definite constructive campaign to place before the British public some real knowledge of and appreciation for New Zealand's dairy industry'.[31] The films were shown at trade demonstrations in cities such as London, Glasgow and Liverpool, and they were pitched at the female consumer because women were responsible for food and feeding families. With the end of the War Commandeer in 1921 and the return to a free market, New Zealand dairy farmers were in crisis. Prices for primary products slumped. Dominion dairy farmers had to promote themselves to British consumers because the British government no longer wanted to boost production to ensure a maximum supply of milk for imperial defence. Farmers' survival depended on responding quickly to the loss of protection that the imperial war economy had provided. Exposed to the winds of the global marketplace, New Zealand sought a united Empire with preferential trade within its borders and was sorely disappointed by the United Kingdom's opposition to imperial preference. Instead it turned to a domestic imperialism: it strove to induce British housewives to give preference to the 'pure quality foods produced in their own Empire overseas'.[32] The Dairy Export Control Board turned to the British woman because, in the words of Lady Burnham, the president of the Society of Women Journalists who visited New Zealand in 1925 with her husband, Lord Burnham, the head of the Empire Press Union, it was the British woman who held the 'house-keeping purse'.[33]

New Zealand dairy farmers realised, like Canadian grain growers, that 'they had to capture minds as well as markets':[34] to capture the grocer and the housewife. In 1936 the New Zealand Labour government, new to office, took control of the icon in an effort to help struggling farmers, introduced guaranteed prices, and made direct shipments of milk products to British ports. Government advertising exhibited the same ideals as the Dairy Board's films of the 1920s. 'Health and vitality' from fresh green pasture and sunshine was the keynote theme. It encapsulated what politicians and farmers imagined to be their advantage in this dependent relationship, whereby 90 per cent of New Zealand's produce travelled to Britain. That it was 'Carried in British ships – manned by British Seamen' denoted both dependence and empire loyalty. The publicity reminded the British housewife that it was better to buy from kin, while sunshine and fresh green pasture gave New Zealand butter its 'unique body and health building properties'.[35]

Nutrition

The representation shared in New Zealand and London was that New Zealand by stocking Britain's larder would produce better British. Ann Stoler has suggested that the Empire became a key 'site' in the production of discourse about European bodies rather than merely a source of contrasts for what a healthy body signified.[36] The argument here is that New Zealand, which imagined itself as part of an imperial community, was a principal site for ideas about a healthy body politic composed of healthy British bodies, and that this reinforced the Britishness of settler identity. In 1925 the eugenically-minded Committee of Inquiry into Mental Defectives and Sexual Offenders said as much in its judgement that: 'It has rightly been decided that this should be not only a "white man's country," but as completely British as possible. We ought to make every effort to keep the stock sturdy and strong, as well as racially pure'.[37] Consistent with this conception, New Zealanders argued that to rear children on 'good New Zealand milk' would secure first-class – white – citizens not only for New Zealand, but for Britain and her Empire/Commonwealth. This idea developed strongly in the inter-war period when agricultural as well as child welfare officials hastened to use what became known as the newer knowledge of nutrition to promote the superiority of New Zealand's dairy products 'in building up a strong constitutioned, virile race'.[38]

For health professionals, exporters, advocates of domestic science and mothercraft, milk became an essential food for growing children, and a medicine to counter racial degeneracy. Sam Adshead has explained that consumerism is more than consumption: it is consumption directed by mentalité: it is mind mattering.[39] If we apply this insight to milk and consumerism in the first half of the twentieth century, it underscores that the consumption of milk was directed by the idea that children mattered. Babies, children and mothers mattered politically because healthy children equated to a healthy nation and vigorous Empire.

Milk, the essential food

Some background is helpful on the enhanced value of child life and health which reinforced medical and agricultural scientific theories about milk's potential for moulding national and imperial physique. The value of the white child, economic and emotional, was transforming from the late nineteenth century.[40] This could be seen in the historic fertility decline in English-speaking countries which signalled fundamental changes in the family and polity, while the birth rate scare that erupted in response elevated further the place of the child in the public mind and in national and imperial anxieties. But it was the First World War, and the grief associated with its violence and the universal 'great sacrifice' of the most able-bodied and dear young men that prompted the growth of the international infant welfare movement, first to 'repair the war wastage', and second to produce 'stronger children, and a fitter race'. 'Long Live King Baby!' became the cry.[41]

Infant mortality rates provided one set of evidence for milk's worth as a body builder. Infant mortality rates served as the yardstick of achievement for campaigns to save baby life and improve national physique. Infant mortality rates were particularly important to New Zealand, for its reputation in health, and especially because it aspired to be a world model for producing the best type of 'His Majesty the Baby'. New Zealand boasted that it had the lowest white infant death rate in the world. I have considered elsewhere the claims by infant health leaders, with New Zealand's Dr Truby King to the forefront, that it was because of infant welfare that infant mortality declined. The point here is the mythology's strength in New Zealand, which likes to be a world model and to invoke 'experiment'.

That the local Plunket Society was portrayed as unique when it was part of an international infant welfare movement demonstrates how culture is a collection, because the way things are put together helps define national cultures. Infant welfare schemes everywhere were shaped by local environments, personalities and politics.[42] Their distinctiveness lay in their indigenous adaptations and manner of piecing together of ideas and practices, more than in the pieces assembled; and in this distinctiveness rested much of their appeal to those engaged in the politics of identity. For many of Truby King's devotees his words held the weight of prophecy because the Truby King 'system' enjoyed patronage at the highest imperial levels. The evident comprehensiveness of infant welfare services in a small country also impressed nations overseas and reinforced the belief that New Zealand was a healthy place to bring up children.[43]

Baby milk

Infant feeding was the focus of the infant welfare movement's drive to lower infant mortality, and milk was synonymous with infant feeding and nourishment, whether given by the mother or the cow. Traditionally, breast milk was essential for infant survival, and infant welfare emphasised the 'transcendent importance' of breast feeding.[44] But as cow's milk entered the global economy, it joined mother's milk as an essential food for infants. In infant welfare edicts, fresh cow's milk provided the best substitute for the milk of a healthy mother, provided it was modified to resemble human milk by being diluted and sweetened, and provided it was 'pure', that is, clean (there was debate as to whether 'pure' meant pasteurised or unpasteurised, as we shall see).[45] Milk from the cow, pure or impure, pasteurised or boiled, fresh or dried, received a fillip from infant welfare schemes, which aimed both to educate mothers in infant care, and to secure a supply of safe milk for the bottle-fed baby. A good mother, while not obliged to breast-feed, had to shun patent foods, condensed milk and 'pieces' from the adults' table. The feeding of children demanded scientific precision.[46] Child nutrition informed by the laws of nature as prescribed by science was the essence of the nation's health.

This message about the vital role of infant feeding with the right sort of milk placed a considerable onus on mothers, as Truby King admonished Australians in the 1920s: 'The problem of right or wrong feeding and nutrition in early infancy is the main determinant of the health and fitness of the being throughout life, and largely determines the fate of the race.'[47] The aim was to win back mothers to have confidence in breast feeding, or if not to use cow's milk modified to conform approximately to human milk: in New Zealand, 'humanised' milk, that is, cow's milk adapted by American methods of percentage feeding to resemble as closely as possible the milk of the average healthy mother. Ironically, artificial formulas and associated rules became the standard, rather than 'Nature's Milk Recipes'. In an era of behaviourism bent on instilling order and self-control, it was easier to fit an individual baby to a regimen and lines on growth charts than to fit feeding formulas to a baby.[48]

Medical input was necessary for milk to be a medicine as desired by scientific farmers, financiers and health experts. Milk from women was not enough to make men strong; racial strength required the guiding hand of nutritional science. For mothers to produce 'not only a fine fat baby', but a 'fine useful man' called for the new science of 'mothercraft'.[49] New Zealand had an advantage in the international race to educate nurses and mothers in mothercraft with its 'Karitane' (Truby King) baby hospitals and mothercraft homes. The most famous was the Mothercraft Training Centre in London, whose patron was the Duchess of York. While the baby could be a king, contemporary gendered language suggested that the king (future queen) was like any other baby. The association of Royalty with babies represented one way in which the Royal Family had begun to refashion itself, at the behest of classes in the white Dominions who needed to believe in the certainty and security symbolised by the British Crown in a period of anxieties, including that about the character of future citizens. In the Dominions many young mothers were impressed by the idea that the regime advertised as used by Royalty had to be worth a try, while New Zealand methods which adapted international ideas were re-exported to produce better babies for the British Empire.

So was New Zealand milk. Baby food companies offer further evidence of colonialism. There is a direct connection between the rise of Glaxo, the multinational pharmaceutical company, and New Zealand's place in the Empire. Joseph Nathan and Company, a Jewish family firm of New Zealand merchants, began Glaxo in a tiny country town in the early 1900s with the aim of supplying dried milk to the United Kingdom. Exporting dried milk solved the problem of surplus skimmed milk in New Zealand dairy factories; and it also solved a problem for infant welfare authorities in England, anxious to secure safe milk for bottle-fed infants. Sir George Newman, a British infant welfare leader and Chief Medical Officer to the Board of

Education, assisted Glaxo's entry to the British market by supervising early infant feeding trials with the New Zealand dried milk in English cities.⁵⁰ The imperial command economy imposed by the First World War firmly established the new dried milk industry. The bulk of Glaxo dried milk manufactured later in the war was purchased by the Imperial Government for soldiers and babies.⁵¹ New Zealand milk in the form of Glaxo, marketed as 'the food that builds bonnie babies', was distributed by municipal infant welfare centres in cities such as Sheffield, Manchester, Salford and Birmingham.⁵²

Glaxo and its construction of New Zealand milk competed directly with the baby mixtures promoted by Truby King and the Plunket Society that were based on fresh cow's milk. The former claimed to be modern, the latter natural, and both to be scientific. From 1927 the Plunket Society joined the pharmaceuticals industry with its Karitane Products, which nurses prescribed to mothers for weaned babies. Karilac – milk sugar – and Kariol – an emulsion of fats and oils – turned cow's milk into an essential food for the baby, by humanising it. Transformed by Karilac and Kariol, cow's milk became a medicine to prevent sickness and death in infants. An infant welfare promotional booklet from the 1940s showed the schoolgirl, the future mother and nurse, in uniform and veil, making up a feeding mixture using Karitane Products as part of her lessons in mothercraft. These essential accessories were a logical extension of Truby King's conviction of rightness. Ironically their supply created demand for substitutes for mother's milk. Glaxo and Karitane Products, both developed in New Zealand, illustrate the competition for control of the icon of imperial milk in infant feeding.

The infant feeding row in the 1920s and 1930s over dried milk and the protein content of the baby's feeding bottle, which I have discussed elsewhere, resulted because feeding the baby *mattered*. When rhetoric resounded about 'His Majesty the Baby', technology, economic linkages, nutritional developments and medicine joined to focus on the child and infant diets. The infant feeding row manifested the baby's entrance to the 'body politic'.⁵³

School milk

Heights and weights provided more evidence for milk's nutritive value as a body builder. Anthropometric surveys suggested New Zealand children were taller and heavier than British children, and slightly taller than Americans and Australians. New Zealand children were heavier than Australian children, though the differences in average heights were insignificant. It was especially important to be better than Australians because New Zealand and Australia were rivals for the title of 'social laboratory', contesting their reputations in social experiment, health policy and sport. The New Zealand evidence from school medical inspections of height and weight gain appeared to vindicate the marketing claims for superior grass and cows, as well as New Zealand parentage and the work of the Plunket Society.⁵⁴ There were parallels of Australasian children with the ANZACs, the soldiers in the Great War who literally looked down on the British. Such evidence, revisited by cliometricians practising anthropometric history, indicates that the increase in heights in the Western world, most rapid in the twentieth century, relates to improved child nutrition. Associated with this increase in heights (a measure of net nutritional status) was a nutritional transition whereby animals rather than grain became the chief source of protein.[55]

Moving from the bottle-fed infant to the cup-drinking child: cow's milk, bottled and pasteurised, became an essential food for the pre-school child and the school child, as the emphasis in health policy shifted from survival to all-round child development by the 1930s. Milk, scientifically processed as a medicine, was promoted as the food most likely to improve children's nutritional status.[56] In the language of recipe books and prescriptive manuals milk was 'first on the list of protective foods'[57] which helped resistance, especially to tuberculosis, and prevented defects in teeth and tonsils which were major concerns from the 1920s to the 1940s. Milk could be a medicine in two ways: as a preventive medicine which ensured children grew straight and strong, and a therapy to build up the weak and repair wasted frames.[58]

From 1924 nutrition classes for children with subnormal nutrition began as part of the campaign for racial improvement. In classes and in health camps, 'health laws' were insisted on, their educational emphasis indicated by placards of milk bottles displaying the message 'eat more milk'.[59] Medical surveys in the United Kingdom by Drs Corry Mann and Boyd Orr in the late 1920s only served to justify New Zealand convictions that to 'eat more milk' increased children's heights and weights.[60] Milk marketing capitalised on both the switch in Western diets to animal protein and its perceived value for building children's bodies, and on the discovery of vitamins. There is evidence of consumerism at work in that vitamins, which were initially called '*accessory* food factors', became *essentials* for human growth and development.[61] New Zealanders were quick to take up British nutritional research; *The NZ Dairy Produce Exporter* publicised in 1925:

> Scientists have stated that it is the presence of these vitamines in milk and its products that has caused the people of the Western Hemisphere who use milk products to have advanced in stature and civilisation beyond the people of the Eastern Hemisphere.[62]

Milk was the 'Master Carpenter' which built and repaired muscles, bones, teeth and nerve cells, a message promoted by home science textbooks into the 1950s.[63]

An advertisement, 'Miss my school milk? I wouldn't be so foolish', depicted a muscular youth downing a glass of milk as part of his weight training.[64] The youth with his milk regime represented New Zealand's answer to Popeye the sailorman, the cartoon character created by E. C. Segar in 1929 who encouraged children to eat spinach. Spinach was no use without milk. By this time – the 1950s – calcium had joined vitamins and 'body-building protein' as scientific evidence of milk's nutritional superiority. Milk was for muscles. The advertisement made this clear: 'Choose A or Z, it matters not, When A's for athlete, Z's for zest; To improve in sport and keep quite fit, Use MILK FOR DRINK, for milk is best.' A fellow who wanted to succeed in sport, or to be 'proud of his build', needed to drink more milk. Scientists had 'proved' that boys and girls needed at least six glasses of milk a day 'to build their bones and help control their muscles'. At this time, milk was being constructed as masculine rather than feminine, as a body-builder. Recollections from the 1940s and 1950s confirm the increasing association of milk with masculinity: it was promoted and used as a sports beverage. Boys carried crates of school milk; and boys had two bottles, whereas girls had one bottle.[65]

The state became the supplier of milk to school children because it was believed that the child as citizen required milk, the most important food, at the very moment that the farmer needed support after the Depression. Internationally there was a worldwide preoccupation with food in the 1930s. The League of Nations urged member countries to institute nutrition inquiries and put milk consumption on the agenda for world agricultural and economic policy. It set a new optimum consumption standard of 1½ to 2 pints (1 litre) daily from the age of two in order to promote and foster optimum child health and development: the 'optimum diet' provided for 'full development of the individual . . . and for the prevention of latent states of malnutrition'.[66] The optimum had become the norm, influenced by the idea that science could better nature.

It was one thing for the League of Nations to recommend a standard for milk consumption that reflected raised standards of health and new scientific optimisms, and another for a country to make changes. Australia responded to the call for nutrition inquiries by setting up an Advisory Council on Nutrition in 1936 which investigated Australian food habits. It found that the problem was with the nutrition of the young child, not nutrition in general.[67] New Zealand on the other hand responded with a national school milk scheme in 1937 and followed this with a series of government nutrition inquiries, beginning with a dietary survey of basic wage-earners in 1939. A survey of Maori diets followed in the 1940s which showed that Maori children drank even less milk, on average, than European children did.[68] Earlier depression surveys of child health by school medical officers and teachers convinced them that 'a milk ration [was] the biggest single influence in improving the nutrition of the children.'[69] The local interpretation of the world emphasis on the young child prioritised school milk because New Zealand's first Labour government assumed control of the icon under the Primary Products Marketing Act 1936, launched a renewed push into the British export market and proceeded to boost demand for milk at home. School milk was introduced nationally, first to benefit the dairy farmer and, second, child health by making the child the emergency consumer who stood to benefit from being one.[70]

From March 1937 a half pint of pasteurised bottled milk a day was available, free, to all children at primary school and kindergarten, and where desired, at secondary school. Where it was impracticable to obtain pasteurised bottled milk schools could resort to malted milk powder for cocoa. School milk was not distinctive to New Zealand. As in so much else in social policy, the idea was imported from England. But the way things are assembled shapes national cultures and identity formation. New Zealand school milk mediated emerging identities within the Welfare State. The half pint bottle of milk a day came, with Plunket, to signify that New Zealand was a healthy place to bring up children. It was supplied free to schools for 30 years, until 1967, when the government dismantled the scheme at the request of Education Boards.

Good and bad milk

The point is that 'good New Zealand milk' was for Britain and so the export industry was regulated, graded and inspected. The milk drunk by New Zealanders encountered no such checks; *bad* milk was a likely prospect. The Second World War compounded the problems since New Zealand was once again 'filling Britain's war-time larder'.[71] The war exposed that two separate markets existed, British and local, with different standards, a state of affairs which had not changed since the beginning of the century. Difficulties with school milk exposed the deficiencies in supply. School milk grew warm because it was not kept refrigerated. Children disliked the taste, which some attributed to pasteurisation, they disliked the cream on top of the milk and some could not drink a full half pint. School milk was never universal; it did not reach isolated settlements; and in schools supplied with milk the consumption rate was 60 per cent.[72] While 'good' milk, which included school milk, was a food and a medicine, bad milk could convey disease and so was to be feared. The New Zealand public had long been advised to 'drink more milk' but many remained suspicious that it might be diseased into the 1950s.[73]

The state only heeded consumer protest in the Second World War, when wartime interest in people's sustenance combined with public outcry to provoke the establishment of a commission of inquiry into the town milk supply in 1943, and a Milk Act based on its findings in 1944. The Milk Commission was appointed to inquire into the milk supply for the four main cities, Auckland, Wellington, Christchurch and Dunedin, because there had been so many complaints about the poor quality of milk and serious shortages in the early 1940s.[74] Bad milk and insufficient quantity had long been a problem because New Zealand dairy farmers put export requirements first. The Second World War threw into sharp relief the discrepancies between bad milk for New Zealand consumers and good milk for the Empire overseas. There were three catalysts for the milk inquiry in 1943–4. First was the demand generated by the British market in the war, which echoed the pressure exerted by the British government in the First World War to provide food for Britain. Second was the new market generated by the presence of American troops in New Zealand during the Pacific War, who demanded milk and milk shakes; and third the school milk scheme, which invited supply problems.

Shortcomings varied by region because there was no national milk policy for domestic milk; this was left to local government and communities. Wellington, the capital city, had a municipal milk supply in terms of centralised treatment from 1919 and distribution from 1922 which provided a model for Delhi in India. In Christchurch, by contrast, free enterprise reigned. As late as 1950 pasteurised milk comprised 24 per cent of milk sold in Christchurch, the lowest proportion in New Zealand, whereas pasteurised milk in Wellington comprised 81 per cent and in Auckland 94 per cent of the market. Provincial towns in dairy farming areas also had high per centages of pasteurised milk because of their connections to the export industry, but nationally the per centage was a mere 61 per cent.[75]

Many complaints in the 1940s came from women as consumers. Women's agency was important in promoting the scientific, professional view that milk was a valuable food, indispensable for children, and in lobbying at the same time for means to prevent disease in milk. The New Zealand Women's Food Value League was one such group of educated female consumers who were enthusiastic about nutritional science and active in the voluntary sector.[76] It campaigned for a woman to represent the welfare of women and children in milk policy when the public inquiry of 1944 exposed its failures. Under the Milk Act 1944 the government appointed a Central Milk Council as a watchdog body. The sole woman member of the Milk Council from 1945, and the only medical member, was Dr Muriel Bell, who was appointed by the Minister of Health to represent the welfare of women and children. Dr Bell was still active on the Milk Board when she died in 1974. The first woman academic in the University of Otago's Faculty of Medicine (as lecturer in physiology) and the first Nutrition Officer in the Department of Health from 1940, a post created to address wartime anxieties about feeding the nation, Muriel Bell held two posts at once, of research and advice, for over 20 years, as state nutritionist and honorary Director of Nutrition Research at the Otago Medical School. At the time she was not supported by the medical establishment who were less knowledgeable about nutrition, especially when compared to women domestic science graduates from the School of Home Science at the University of Otago. For many years Muriel Bell was the main figure in nutrition in New Zealand and one of her many goals was a safe, cheap milk supply.[77]

It bothered Bell that New Zealanders, like Australians and Britons, drank relatively little milk (though more than the British). This was not simply because they were deterred by dirty cowyards, smell and the lingering perception that milk was diseased. From the household point of view, liquid milk was a non-essential. Families supplied it as an accessory side dish, as bread and butter, scones and cream, or milk in tea, and commonly had butter

92   *Philippa Mein Smith*

and cream rather than milk to drink. There was apathy to milk in rural districts where people saw too much of it, while for some it was a luxury; the urban poor did not drink it. In the Depression, the National Council of Women observed that people were urged not to use condensed milk but often they had no alternative because of the price.[78] Evidently milk was price- as well as income-elastic.[79] In consumption trends there was a slight increase from the 1890s to the 1930s from 280 to 340 mls a person a day (from under one-half pint to five-eighths of a pint). Liquid milk consumption was the same in the 1890s as in the 1990s, but the demand curve has shifted.[80] Until the 1940s price was a factor: for 30 years, from 1945 to 1976, the state subsidised milk and fixed the price to the consumer at 4c a pint. Per capita consumption peaked in the 1950s coincident with the promotion through schools and since then there has been a change in tastes.

Be British: eat raw milk

The city of Christchurch offers a case study of how milk represented mind mattering and so became a subject of political controversy. It offers an historical example of the layering of identities and local variation because its citizens used contests for resources in the market for town milk to assert regional identity over national identity. In 1952 Christchurch was the only city which had not opted for pasteurised milk and the associated requirement of centralised milk treatment. Christchurch has always been suspicious of policy from Wellington, and showed this when confronted with the prospect of compulsorily pasteurised milk in the 1940s and 1950s. In the ensuing controversy, Christchurch raw milk advocates invoked their Britishness and promoted their city as a bastion of supposedly English virtues.

For cow's milk to have value as a children's food, paradoxically it first had to be restored to purity.[81] In 1906 the Christchurch City Council followed international trends when it decided that the town milk supply had to be reformed for milk to be publicised as a body-builder and a medicine to prevent disease, rather than as a source of diseases such as infant diarrhoea and tuberculosis.[82] The city also heeded specific national concerns that the milk consumed by New Zealanders was not graded and inspected like the milk exported as dairy products. Dr J. M. Mason, one of the new sanitarians and head of New Zealand's Department of Public Health (established in 1901), and J. A. Kinsella, the Canadian-born Dairy Commissioner in the Department of Agriculture, voiced these concerns nationally. While Kinsella instituted the system of grading for export, Mason envisaged a municipal pasteurising factory in each town, the equivalent of the export butter factory. Both asserted that milk was often transformed from an 'ideal food for children' into an 'agent for ill-health and death'.[83] Drawing on international literature, Christchurch contemplated a municipal milk supply, the main models for which were Buenos Aires and Johannesburg because of Kinsella's influence. He had inspected Buenos Aires' central pasteurised milk depots, while he had worked for the Transvaal government before he moved to New Zealand, assisting the Johannesburg City Council to prepare regulations for the city milk trade and vendors to form a cooperative milk company.[84]

Despite these early moves, Christchurch declined to act for 40 years until forced to do so by the commission of inquiry into urban milk in 1944. There was debate about the milk supply after 1906 in which pasteurisation proved the stumbling block. While the medical profession were divided on the issue, so were the milk lobby and suspicious consumers who perceived raw milk as the ideal, and pasteurisation as unnatural, and a means to disguise bad milk. The City Council opted for 'natural' milk delivered pure and protected from sunlight.[85] In 1927 it revisited the idea of a municipal milk supply when a committee of doctors undertook a bacteriological survey of milk with the view to introducing a scheme like Wellington's, but political economy was influencing local identity and the City Council balked at the state socialism suggested by pasteurisation. A price war in the depression prompted another round of deferrals, despite complaints from vendors about unfair competition from insanitary suppliers.[86]

The city's milk supply was left to private enterprise until the wartime Labour government and its Central Milk Council intervened nationally from 1945, perceiving pasteurised milk as a matter of public health and public interest. In Christchurch, a public row over raw versus pasteurised milk proved a major reason for the insistence that market forces should predominate, because raw milk represented the other side of the coin of deregulation in the milk market. The row revealed more than dominant conservative politics. Christchurch consumers demanded the right of choice between raw milk, represented as 'fresh', and milk which was not pasteurised 'BUT COOKED'.[87] Taste was important because pasteurised milk tasted different and Christchurch consumers were accustomed to the flavour of unpasteurised milk. Crucially, however, raw milk advocates saw themselves as 'fighting to preserve . . . freedom and the British way of life'.[88] Local small businessmen, suspicious of government interference and the growth of big business suggested by the pasteurisation plant, invoked the idea that fresh, raw milk was a health-giving food which conferred 'natural immunity'; and then equated naturalness with Britishness.[89] The right to choose 'fresh' milk became constructed as a matter of British identity.

Christchurch was established as an English settlement in 1850 according to the theory of systematic colonisation which aimed to transplant a slice of rural England to the colonies. Belief in Englishness peaked about the time of the city's centennial in 1950 and informed the milk controversy, while the dispute over raw milk offered a vehicle for the expression of this English identity. It was important for Christchurch to be more English than the rest of New Zealand because the city was busy regilding its foundation myths, while the general climate was still one of empire loyalty. The association of raw milk with Britishness through what it represented in the form of right of choice, fighting for democracy, freedom and nature, occurred at a moment of renewed emphasis on British values because of patriotism in the Second World War and the local drive to be the most and best of British.[90] It was this assertion of identity which prompted the city to diverge from the national and international trend and decide against complete pasteurisation despite state public health imperatives.

The milk controversy came to a head in 1953 when the Medical Officer of Health, responsible to the state Health Department, tried to introduce compulsory pasteurisation with the authority of the Minister of Health using powers under the Health Act. Public outcry prompted the instruction's withdrawal. In 1954 the raw milk lobby formed into the Milk Consumers' Protection Association, provoked by a transfer of milk rounds in middle-class suburbs to pasteurised milk vendors. One consumer insisted on her democratic rights to 'raw pure milk'; she preferred 'live bodies rather than dead bodies' in her milk and would have 'no man or group of men dictating what her family or grandchildren should drink'.[91] Right of choice remained the issue. The 1954 Royal Visit was a reminder of freedoms: why should politicians deny these over milk?[92] The result was a rezoning of milk rounds so that consumers had a choice of raw or pasteurised milk and of vendor.[93]

It took a disease emergency, first over tuberculosis and second over undulant fever in the late 1950s for the city's milk to be compulsorily pasteurised. The state used its emergency powers to protect public health and directed that all milk in Christchurch be pasteurised until such time as the milk supply was disease-free. Bacteriological tests showed that 70 per cent of herds supplying Christchurch's two bulk treatment stations were infected with brucellosis in 1957, while tuberculosis and undulant fever organisms were found in raw milk. Some large herds supplying Christchurch milk were infected with tuberculosis by as much as 50 per cent in 1958.[94] The issue was settled late in 1961 once the disease scare was effectively dealt with. Thus the milk supply was not generally safe in New Zealand cities until after the Second World War, and in Christchurch not until the 1960s.[95]

Shifting identities

'We are what we eat' took on particular meaning for Christchurch consumers in relation to milk. This case study demonstrates how 'what people eat expresses who and what they are, to themselves and to others'.[96] Through insisting on raw milk, Christchurch stalwarts perceived themselves as even more British than the rest of New Zealand which, collectively, still assumed this ethnic label. In the process they thwarted public health objectives.

From the 1960s, children ceased to be so central to discourse about milk's body-building properties. A study of milk promotion material shows how state interest shifted from babies, to young children, to adolescents and adults. Human capital arguments for building children's bodies ceased to be paramount. School milk was discontinued, to the distress of Dr Muriel Bell who urged politicians not to take risks with children's health, citing the surveys by Dr Corry Mann and local studies of height and weight gain to no avail.[97] Bell was early to recognise the risks of osteoporosis and thought the benefits of the school milk scheme would not be known until the 1980s, suspecting they would be greatest for girls.[98] Milk continued to be promoted as 'our best single food', and the most important for public health.[99] But with new nutritional knowledge milk was no longer just a children's food; it became a food for adults as part of a balanced diet. State-sponsored advertising in the 1960s stated 'everything tastes better with cream'.[100]

The target moved to men, who were advised to drink milk not beer, to improve their work productivity and reduce accidents. Milk, the ultimate feminine food, had become masculine. As for boys in the 1950s, the message – 'I was pint sized' suggested that milk consumption promoted muscles and masculinity. Supply by the state made it possible for milk to assume the qualities appropriate to a man rather than a woman and a mother. There had been a shift not only in the targeted age group but in gendered identities: from state protection of babies to state protection of adult men. For milk to be presented as a medicine for women to prevent osteoporosis and ageing by building up calcium deposits had to wait until the 1980s. The feminisation of consumption accompanied the changing position of women in the late twentieth century and the feminisation of ageing that resulted from longer life spans.

A core theme of this essay is that milk was constructed as a medium for 'building Britons' and layers of British identity in New Zealand. Infant and child welfare experts, school doctors, women trained in domestic science and nutritionists were key participants in this process. So were dairy farmers keen to promote their product in a system of guaranteed markets which continued New Zealand's dependency upon Britain until the United Kingdom turned towards Europe from the 1960s. For as long as Britain thought imperially, New Zealand remained ostensibly British.

An analysis of milk and its transformation into an imperial icon of health, informed by the social history of medicine, illuminates how New Zealand's settler identity has changed over the twentieth century. This study has plotted the transitions in good New Zealand milk from a means to build robust babies for empire, to an essential food supplied by the state to make children strong, to a drink subsidised by the state to improve the strength of adult men. Medical constructions of children's bodies in the interests of racial strength and the privileging of the male body occurred in the context of New Zealand's enduring imperial ties, economically, to the United Kingdom. Milk became refeminised when it was no longer for building Britons. The notion of milk as a body-builder itself represented a form of cultural imperialism, derived not from the metropole but from the Dominion of New Zealand. The 'Empire' created in New Zealand by milk to provide food, soldiers and babies for Britain was not imposed: New Zealand, that is, the New Zealand created by settler capitalism, was a source of the images, a site of the image-making and of associated, self-generated, identities.

Britishness lost its appeal for shaping a collective identity when Britain joined Europe. New Zealand abruptly ceased to be the Empire's dairy farm. Its settler society and identity was 'unsettled' with the enforced restructuring of the economy, repositioning in the world and a developing sense of indigenous identities shaped by new cultural and political relations.[101] In a deregulated economy and changed society the product, milk, has diversified. But the icon, milk, the medicine and body-builder, maintains its tie with New Zealandness. There is a continuity in the clean, green, healthy, image projected in advertisements and in New Zealanders' nostalgic responses to such imagery. How others see us continues to affect how we see ourselves.

Notes

1 W. K. Hancock edited the official British histories of the Second World War and wrote the classic Australian work, *Australia* (London: Benn, 1930). For his views on imperial history, see W. K. Hancock, 'Agenda for the Study of British Imperial Economy 1850–1950', *Journal of Economic History*, Vol. XIII, no. 3, 1953.
2 NZ High Commission, Canberra, correspondence with author, May 1996.
3 On ideals in advertisements, see G. R. Lealand, *A Foreign Egg in Our Nest? American Popular Culture in New Zealand* (Wellington: Victoria University Press, 1988), pp. 6–9.
4 Avner Offer, *The First World War: An Agrarian Interpretation* (Oxford: Clarendon Press, 1989), p. 137.
5 See Gil Docking with additions by Michael Dunn, *Two Hundred Years of New Zealand Painting*, rev. edn (Auckland: David Batemen, 1990).
6 The Statute of Westminster was passed by the Imperial Parliament in 1931. It afforded independent sovereign status to the white British Dominions: Australia, New Zealand, Canada, South Africa and Ireland.
7 A. L. Stoler, *Race and the Education of Desire: Foucault's History of Sexuality and the Colonial Order of Things* (Durham, NC and London: Duke University Press, 1995), p. 200.
8 Culture refers to a shared set of values or beliefs, and ways of living, while identity refers to defining the self, including in relation to agreed values. A. Pagden and N. Canny have usefully encapsulated the relation between culture and identity in their observation that the 'possession of an identity also presupposes the existence of a shared set of cultural values'. 'Afterword: From Identity to Independence', in N. Canny and A. Pagden (eds), *Colonial Identity in the Atlantic World, 1500–1800* (Princeton, NJ: Princeton University Press, 1987), p. 269.
9 In 1973, the writer Frank Sargeson published a memoir which revealed how white (Pakeha) New Zealanders internalised this image of the Empire's dairy farm: 'looking back across the patchwork of farmland', he wrote, 'I saw the crowns of a group of cabbage trees superimposed against an immense blue ribbon of sea: it was all very well for the Empire's dairy farm to be momentarily annihilated, but I could not help being suspicious of the involuntarily romantic images of tropical islands and palms that it was immediately replaced by.' F. Sargeson, *Once is Enough: A Memoir* (Wellington: A. H. & A. W. Reed, 1973), p. 41.
10 Donald Denoon, *Settler Capitalism: The Dynamics of Dependent Development in the Southern Hemisphere* (Oxford: Clarendon Press, 1983).
11 S. A. M. Adshead, *Material Culture in Europe and China, 1400–1800* (Basing-

stoke and London: Macmillan, 1997). See also D. W. Curtin and L. M. Heldke (eds), *Cooking, Eating, Thinking: Transformative Philosophies of Food* (Bloomington and Indianapolis: Indiana University Press, 1992).
12 Francis McKee, 'The Popularisation of Milk as a Beverage during the 1930s', in David F. Smith (ed.), *Nutrition in Britain: Science, Scientists and Politics in the Twentieth Century* (Routledge: London and New York, 1997), pp. 123–41. This association with purity and life was cross-cultural, as images attest of the Indian god Krishna as a baby, fed by the cow-mother.
13 Adshead, *Material Culture in Europe and China*, p. 1.
14 Recent works on the international infant welfare movement include Valerie Fildes, Lara Marks and Hilary Marland (eds), *Women and Children First: International Maternal and Infant Welfare, 1870–1945* (London and New York: Routledge, 1992); Alisa Klaus, *Every Child a Lion: The Origins of Maternal and Infant Health Policy in the United States and France, 1890–1920* (Ithaca, NY and London: Cornell University Press, 1993); Cynthia Comacchio, '*Nations Are Built of Babies': Saving Ontario's Mothers and Children 1900–1940* (Montreal: McGill-Queen's University Press, 1993); Lara V. Marks, *Metropolitan Maternity: Maternal and Infant Welfare Services in Early Twentieth Century London* (Amsterdam and Atlanta, GA: Rodopi, 1996); Richard A. Meckel, *Save the Babies: American Public Health Reform and the Prevention of Infant Mortality, 1850–1929* (Baltimore, MD: Johns Hopkins University Press, 1990); Philippa Mein Smith, *Mothers and King Baby: Infant Survival and Welfare in an Imperial World: Australia 1880–1950* (Basingstoke and London: Macmillan, 1997).
15 Draft of letter by Muriel Bell to *Otago Daily Times*, June 1955, copy in file on milk in schools compiled by Flora Davidson, former nutritionist in the Department of Health. File in possession of J. Reid, Senior Advisor (Food and Nutrition), Ministry of Health, Wellington.
16 This idea has benefited from Stoler, *Race and the Education of Desire*; K. Oliver, 'Nourishing the Speaking Subject: A Psychoanalytic Approach to Abominable Food and Women', in Curtin and Heldke (eds), *Cooking, Eating, Thinking*; and C. Smith-Rosenberg, 'The Body Politics', in Elizabeth Weed (ed.), *Coming to Terms: Feminism, Theory, Politics* (New York: Routledge, 1989).
17 Curtin and Heldke (eds), *Cooking, Eating, Thinking*, p. xiii.
18 These thoughts have been assisted by C. P. Gutierrez, *Cajun Foodways* (Jackson: University Press of Mississippi, 1992), pp. 3–4, 33, 137.
19 F. Truby King, *The Feeding of Plants and Animals* (Wellington: Whitcombe and Tombs, 1905), pp. 5, 6, 8.
20 Truby King promoted his ideas as being true to natural law. But in fact the Truby King 'system' was most unnatural. On Truby King and his rules, see Mein Smith, *Mothers and King Baby*, ch. 4. Other sources include Mary Truby King, *Truby King the Man* (London: Allen & Unwin, 1948); Christina Hardyment, *Dream Babies: Child Care from Locke to Spock* (London: Jonathan Cape, 1983).
21 The term 'fattening human stock' is from Margaret Tennant, *Children's Health, The Nation's Wealth: A History of Children's Health Camps* (Wellington: Bridget Williams Books/Historical Branch, 1994), ch. 2; also P. Mein Smith, *Maternity in Dispute: New Zealand 1920–1939* (Wellington: Government Printer/Historical Branch, 1986), p. 3.
22 S. W. Mintz, *Sweetness and Power* (New York: Penguin Books, 1985), p. xxix.
23 These thoughts have benefited from Mintz, ch. 2, 'Production'.
24 Alfred W. Crosby, *Ecological Imperialism: The Biological Expansion of Europe, 900–1900* (New York: Cambridge University Press, 1986).
25 H. G. Philpott, *A History of the New Zealand Dairy Industry 1840–1935* (Wellington: Government Printer, 1937), p. 12.

26 NZ Dairy Produce Exporter, 25 July 1925, pp. 30–1.
27 W. D. McIntyre, 'Australia, New Zealand, and the Pacific Islands', in *Oxford History of the British Empire*, Vol. 4 (Oxford: OUP, 1999).
28 The films were described at length in the NZ Dairy Produce Exporter, 29 May 1926; quotation from p. 21.
29 Miles Fairburn, *The Ideal Society and Its Enemies: The Foundations of Modern New Zealand Society 1850–1900* (Auckland: Auckland University Press, 1989), p. 29.
30 NZ Dairy Produce Exporter, 29 May 1926, p. 44. The reference to Maori warriors and imperial troops related to the New Zealand Wars of the 1860s. Much of the land confiscated as a result of the wars was used for dairy farming from the 1890s.
31 NZ Dairy Produce Exporter, ibid. The movies coincided with the Dairy Board's attempt to seize control of the marketing of New Zealand dairy products in the United Kingdom. Indeed they were part of this strategy. Between them, the movies contained all the symbols of a British identity in New Zealand as it existed in the 1920s. The fifth film described New Zealand as 'Britain overseas'.
32 NZ Dairy Produce Exporter, 29 August 1925, pp. 18–19. For a cultural studies view of domestic imperialism, see Anne McClintock, *Imperial Leather: Race, Gender and Sexuality in the Colonial Contest* (New York and London: Routledge, 1995).
33 'British Women Favour Empire Grown Products'. Interview with Lady (Viscountess) Burnham, ibid.
34 Offer, *The First World War*, p. 149.
35 Display at London Grocers' Exhibition, AJHR, 1939, H-30, p. 1.
36 Stoler, *Race and the Education of Desire*, pp. 7–11.
37 AJHR, 1925, H-31A, p. 28, cited in Mein Smith, *Maternity in Dispute*, p. 25.
38 W. M. Singleton, Director, Dairy Division, Department of Agriculture, NZ Dairy Produce Exporter, 25 July 1925, p. 30.
39 Adshead, *Material Culture*.
40 On the transformation in the value of the (white, normal) child as the child changed from a worker to a scholar, see Viviana Zelizer, *Pricing the Priceless Child* (New York: Basic Books, 1985), republished 1994. See also Roger Cooter (ed.), *In the Name of the Child: Health and Welfare 1880–1940* (London: Routledge, 1992).
41 Mein Smith, *Mothers and King Baby*, p. 63.
42 See, for example, Mein Smith, *Mothers and King Baby*, ch. 6.
43 Ibid., ch. 4.
44 Ibid., p. 93.
45 In the Christchurch controversy over raw vs. pasteurised milk.
46 See Mein Smith, *Mothers and King Baby*, pp. 66–7 and ch. 4. On 'scientific' infant feeding in the United States, see Rima D. Apple, *Mothers and Medicine: A Social History of Infant Feeding, 1890–1950* (Madison, WI: University of Wisconsin Press, 1987).
47 Truby King to ed., *Argus*, Melbourne, 17 February 1923, cited in Mein Smith, *Mothers and King Baby*, p. 93.
48 Mein Smith, *Mothers and King Baby*, p. 103; see also Helen May, *The Discovery of Early Childhood: The Development of Services for the Care and Education of Very Young Children, Mid Eighteenth Century Europe to Mid Twentieth Century New Zealand* (Auckland: Auckland University Press/Bridget Williams Books, 1997), p. 145.
49 E. Pritchard, *Infant Education*, 2nd edn (London: Henry Kimpton, 1920), p. 64, cited in Mein Smith, *Mothers and King Baby*, p. 102. The word 'mothercraft' was invented ca. 1910. Anna Davin, 'Imperialism and Motherhood', *History*

Workshop, issue 5, Spring 1978, p. 34, and Deborah Dwork, *War is Good for Babies and Other Young Children: A History of the Infant and Child Welfare Movement in England 1898–1918* (London and New York: Tavistock, 1987).
50 R. P. T. Davenport-Hines and Judy Slinn, *Glaxo: A History to 1962* (Cambridge: Cambridge University Press, 1992), chs 1–2. On Newman, see Dwork, *War is Good for Babies*.
51 Philpott, *A History of the New Zealand Dairy Industry 1840–1935*, pp. 108, 152–61.
52 Davenport-Hines and Slinn, *Glaxo: A History to 1962*, pp. 41–3.
53 On the infant feeding row, see P. Mein Smith, "That Welfare Warfare", in Fildes, Marks and Marland (eds), *Women and Children First*, ch. 11, and *Mothers and King Baby*, ch. 5.
54 Ada G. Paterson and E. Marsden, 'Physical Growth and Mental Attainment: New Zealand Schoolchildren', *Appendices to Journals of the House of Representatives*, hereafter *AJHR*, 1927, H-31, Appendix, pp. 54–63.
55 On the nutritional transition, see D. Grigg, 'The Nutritional Transition in Western Europe', *Journal of Historical Geography*, Vol. 21, no. 3, 1995, pp. 247–61. For a useful essay review of developments in anthropometric history, see Bernard Harris, 'Health, Height, and History: An Overview of Recent Developments in Anthropometric History', *Social History of Medicine*, Vol. 7, no. 2, August 1994, pp. 297–320. Major works in the field include R. W. Fogel, 'Nutrition and the Decline in Mortality since 1700: Some Preliminary Findings', in S. L. Engerman and R. E. Gallman (eds), *Long-Term Factors in American Economic Growth* (Chicago: University of Chicago Press, 1986), pp. 439–555, and R. Floud, K. Wachter and A. Gregory, *Height, Health and History: Nutritional Status in the United Kingdom, 1750–1980* (Cambridge: Cambridge University Press, 1990). For relevant work on Australia, see R. V. Jackson and Mark Thomas, 'Height, Weight, and Wellbeing: Sydney Schoolchildren in the Early Twentieth Century', *Australian Economic History Review*, Vol. XXXV, no. 2, 1995, pp. 39–65.
56 There are numerous examples in Flora Davidson file, Ministry of Health.
57 Department of Health, *Hints on Diet* (Wellington: Government Printer, 1935).
58 Davenport-Hines and Slinn, *Glaxo*, p. 26.
59 Flora Davidson file, Ministry of Health; Tennant, *Children's Health, The Nation's Wealth*, p. 33. Initially subnormal nutrition was determined by clinical judgment of a child's skinniness, pallor and posture. From the 1930s doctors and teachers adopted more 'scientific' (quantitative) tests based on height and weight charts, and in New Zealand the measure for child malnutrition became 10 per cent below the ideal weight for age line, as used in Toronto. School medical officers used the Toronto scale to make an age-height-weight survey of New Zealand children in 1934, H. C. D. Somerset, *Child Nutrition in a Rural Community* (Wellington: NZ Council for Educational Research, 1941), Studies in Education no. 6, pp. 15–16.
60 On these British/Scottish trials to test the efficacy of milk, see McKee, 'The Popularisation of Milk as a Beverage', pp. 25–6. An early example of imitation of Corry Mann and Orr's trials in New Zealand, among Maori children, is H. B. Turbott and A. F. Rolland, 'The Nutritional Value of Milk. Experimental Evidence from Maori Schoolchildren', *New Zealand Medical Journal*, Vol. 31, 1932, pp. 109–111. Turbott was the local Medical Officer of Health and Rolland the Head Teacher at a rural Native School. They concluded: 'The milk rationing resulted not only in physical improvement judged by gain in height and weight and by improved resistance to disease, but also in improved mental alertness . . . it is certain that milk has a very high nutritive value', ibid., p. 111.
61 On the spectrum of accessory to essential, see Adshead, *Material Culture*.

62 *NZ Dairy Produce Exporter*, 25 July 1925, p. 31. On vitamins and their commercialisation, see Sally M. Horrocks, 'Nutrition Science and the Food and Pharmaceutical Industries in Inter-War Britain', in David F. Smith (ed.), *Nutrition in Britain*, pp. 53–74.
63 An example was the Home Science Scholar's Note Book (Whitcombe and Tombs, 1954).
64 'Milk in Schools', Muriel Bell Papers, MS 1078, Box 1. The advertisement featured in the *New Zealand Trades Alphabet*, 1955, p. 47, and copies were delivered to *ca.* 250,000 schoolchildren. Christchurch City Council, CCC CH 380, vol. 2, c/154, National Archives, Christchurch.
65 Oral testimony, History seminar, University of Canterbury, June 1996.
66 Vera Scantlebury Brown, 'Nutrition of the Pre-School Child', *Medical Journal of Australia*, 30 July 1938, p. 153; Mein Smith, *Mothers and King Baby*, p. 229.
67 Mein Smith, ibid., pp. 222–3; F. W. Clements, *A History of Human Nutrition in Australia* (Melbourne: Longman Cheshire, 1986), Section III.
68 Medical Research Council, *Report of Nutrition Research Committee, 1939–40*, Muriel Bell Papers, MS 1078, Box 1; E. Gregory, P. R. Jackson, E. C. Chambers and E. C. G. McLaughlin, 'New Zealand Dietary Studies I: Dietary Studies of One Hundred and Seventy Families of Varying Occupations', *NZ Medical Journal*, April 1943; E. C. G. McLaughlin, 'New Zealand Dietary Studies II: Dietary Survey among Basic Wage-Earners', *NZ Medical Journal*, August 1943; E. C. G. McLaughlin and I. Wilson, 'New Zealand Dietary Studies III: Dietary Survey among Maoris', *NZ Medical Journal*, April 1945, pp. 1–6. Average daily consumption of milk was 0.7 pint (395 ml), and among Maori, 0.6 pint (342 ml), Muriel E. Bell, 'School Milk in New Zealand', *XIVth International Dairy Congress Proceedings*, Nutrition Section, Vol. 1, 1956, p. 1.
69 H. C. D. Somerset, *Child Nutrition in a Rural Community*, p. 28. Somerset was an exceptional teacher who conducted his own surveys. His wife Gwen Somerset was an expert on early childhood.
70 Muriel Bell to G. A. Q. Lennane, 'Milk in Schools Scheme', 11 February 1961, in Flora Davidson file, Ministry of Health.
71 The British Ministry of Food renewed long-term contracts for all New Zealand's exportable surpluses of dairy products from 1944–8, *AJHR*, 1944, H-30, pp. 3–5. Bulk purchasing arrangements only ceased in 1955.
72 Flora Davidson file, Ministry of Health.
73 See, for example, J. A. Kinsella, 'A Plea for Purer Milk Supply for Human Consumption in our Cities and Towns', unpublished paper, 1906, CCC CH 343/94a, National Archives, Christchurch. Cf. comments in 1948 by Dr Lonie, MOH Palmerston North, Flora Davidson file.
74 Milk Commission, *Report on the Supply of Milk to the Four Metropolitan Areas of Auckland, Wellington, Christchurch, and Dunedin*, *AJHR*, 1944, H-29A.
75 Palmerston North had 90 per cent pasteurised milk, and Gisborne 97 per cent. By comparison, in London in 1942 pasteurised milk comprised 90 per cent of the supply, while in Scotland 44 per cent of town milk was pasteurised. F. B. Smith, *The Retreat of Tuberculosis 1850–1950* (London: Croom Helm, 1988), p. 193. My source for Wellington as a model for Delhi is Ian Catanach.
76 S. Coney, 'New Zealand Women's Food Value League 1937–1948', in A. Else (ed.), *Women Together: A History of Women's Organisations in New Zealand* (Wellington: Daphne Brasell/Historical Branch, 1993), pp. 270–1.
77 P. Mein Smith, 'Muriel E. Bell', *Dictionary of New Zealand Biography*, Vol. 4 (Auckland and Wellington: Auckland University Press/Dept of Internal Affairs, 1998), pp. 47–8; Muriel Bell Papers, MS 1078, Hocken Library. See also D. A. Dow, *Safeguarding the Public Health: A History of the New Zealand Department of Health* (Wellington: Victoria University Press, 1995), pp. 144–6.

78 'Council of Women', *Herald*, 30 April 1934, NCW (Auckland branch), Newspaper Cuttings, MS 879, series 12, box 2, item 155, Auckland Institute and Museum Library.
79 F. Devonport, 'An Enquiry into the Condition of the Liquid Milk Industry in Christchurch', M. Com. (Hons) thesis in Economics, Canterbury University College, 1949.
80 Consumption figures calculated by Flora Davidson, 'Trends in Milk Consumption in New Zealand', unpublished conference paper, Nutrition Society, August 1982, Ministry of Health.
81 See, for example, Meckel, *Save the Babies*; McKee, 'The Popularisation of Milk as a Beverage'.
82 J. A. Kinsella, 'A Plea for a Purer Milk Supply for Human Consumption in our Cities and Towns', unpublished paper, 1906, CCC CH 343/94a, National Archives, Christchurch.
83 *Lyttelton Times*, 19 September 1906, CCC CH 343/94a, National Archives, Christchurch.
84 Kinsella, 'A Plea for a Purer Milk Supply'.
85 Christchurch City Council, Milk Supply, 1906, CH 343/94a, National Archives, Christchurch.
86 Christchurch City Council, *Abattoir, Reserves, Market and Milk Committee Minutes*, 1927–1935, CCC CH 380, c/100 no. 4, c/103 no. 4, National Archives, Christchurch.
87 Christchurch Metropolitan Milk Board, Chairman's Report, 14 June 1954, CCC CH 380, Vol. 2, c/154, National Archives, Christchurch.
88 W. B. Crowley on radio with W. Kennedy, MOH for Christchurch, *Listener*, 7 August 1953, p. 5.
89 Milk Consumers' Protection Association, Deputation to Christchurch Metropolitan Milk Board, Christchurch Metropolitan Milk Board, *Minutes*, 17 June 1957, CCC CH 380, Vol. 2, c/154, National Archives, Christchurch; discussion with J. E. Cookson, whose mother was the Mayoress of Christchurch in the 1940s.
90 The formation of Christchurch identity is analysed in John Cookson and Graeme Dunstall (eds), *Southern Capital: Towards a City Biography 1850-2000* (Christchurch: Canterbury University Press, 2000).
91 Mrs Crowley, Milk Consumers' Protection Association, Deputation to Christchurch Metropolitan Milk Board, Christchurch Metropolitan Milk Board, *Minutes*, 17 June 1957, CCC CH 380, Vol. 2, c/154, National Archives, Christchurch.
92 *Press*, Christchurch, 9 June 1954, p. 9.
93 Ibid. Lobbying the National (conservative) Government was a success to ensure freedom of choice (the MP for Fendalton was the Prime Minister).
94 Christchurch Metropolitan Milk Board, *Minutes*, September 1958–June 1959, February 1960, CCC CH 380, Vol. 2, c/154, Vol. 3, c/155, National Archives, Christchurch.
95 An exception was Wellington because of its early move to pasteurised milk, relative to other New Zealand cities – but not relative to cities overseas.
96 Mintz, *Sweetness and Power*, p. 13, also pp. 3–4.
97 Submission to the Commission of Education by NZ Milk Board regarding School Milk by Muriel E. Bell, and, 'Milk-in-Schools Scheme – A Review', 5 August 1966, Muriel Bell to G. A. Q. Lennane, Director, Division of Child Hygiene, 11 February 1961, Ministry of Health file.
98 Muriel Bell, 'Osteoporosis as a Dietary Problem', *Journal of the NZ Dietetic Association*, Vol. 15, no. 1, June 1961, pp. 13–18.
99 Muriel Bell, 'Milk – Our Best Single Food', *Listener*, 23 May 1941; *AJHR*, 1950, H-31.

100 Posters, Milk Board, Prodn no. 47840/65, Accession no. 140, National Archives, Christchurch.
101 See, for example, Wendy Larner and Paul Spoonley, 'Post-Colonial Politics in Aotearoa/New Zealand', in Daiva Stasiulis and Nira Yuval-Davis (eds), *Unsettling Settler Societies: Articulations of Gender, Race, Ethnicity and Class*, Sage Series on Race and Ethnic Relations, Vol. 11 (London: Sage, 1995), pp. 39–64; Donald Denoon, 'Settler Capitalism Unsettled', *NZ Journal of History*, Vol. 29, no. 2, October 1995, pp. 129–41; and Donald Denoon, Philippa Mein Smith and Marivic Wyndham, *A History of Australia, New Zealand and the Pacific*, Blackwell History of the World Series (Oxford and Malden: MA: Blackwell, 2000), for an extended treatment of the formation of identities in the region.

6 Tropical medicine and colonial identity in northern Australia

Suzanne Parry

The last decades of the twentieth century witnessed a growing interest in the history of European colonialism and its aftermath. Of particular interest in Australia has been impact of colonialism on identity formation.[1] The highly contentious area of the politics of identity has both grown from and been shaped by studies in this area. It is reasonable to assume that all aspects of Australia's colonial past will continue to be of interest, as long as Australian governments remain embroiled in issues of reconciliation, and the welfare of indigenous people is subject to international scrutiny. Adding to the on-going interest in our colonial past are the challenges being mounted to policies of past legislators and administrators in the highest courts of the land. The court challenge, for instance, against the Australian government by the 'stolen generation', which was played out on the eve of the new millennium, has ensured that the politics of identity continue to be of importance to the nation. In that challenge, the legitimacy of actions taken in Australia's colonial past was hotly contested. As many of those involved in the stolen generations court case came to realise, Australia's colonial past was difficult to isolate in either spatial or temporal terms and the ethical, moral and legal principles guiding it proved elusive and difficult to substantiate. Ultimately, the circumstances that allowed the enacting of legislation that made provision for children of mixed Aboriginal descent to be removed from their Aboriginal families, and the policies of its implementation, were seen to be irrelevant and the case was argued on points of law. Nevertheless, an exploration of that past can be meaningful and such is the task of this chapter.

Recognising that ideological positioning and social interactions are multi-faceted, it will be argued that one highly significant element of the colonial past was the identity of the people as it was shaped in time and space. Here the time will be delineated as the first half of the twentieth century and the place as northern Australia and the identity as that shaped by white male settlers. Of particular interest is the role of the discourse of tropical medicine in the shaping of that identity. It will be argued that an important component in the process of identity formation amongst colonisers was to position indigenous people and to thus 'identify' them in particular ways. Issues relating to health were significant in this regard both in tropical and temperate Australia and remain so today. But, as will be argued below, the discourse of tropical medicine, validated through the idealism of scientific discourse, gave particular legitimacy to the positioning of indigenous people. This is not to suggest that the discourse of tropical medicine was *the* most significant factor in shaping a northern identity but that it was *a* factor and its exploration can be instructive of the ways in which the medicalised body became an important signifier of difference between white settlers and indigenous people in northern Australia.

Tropical medicine

The role of colonial medicine in colonialism and identity formation has begun to be explored in recent times and tropical medicine as a political construct is also now receiving attention. Tropical medicine generally, however, has been of interest to historians since its inception and has been through several phases since Patrick Mason first published his book *Tropical Diseases* in 1898. In his 1988 review of the historiography of tropical medicine Roy MacLeod identifies four approaches adopted by historians. The earliest approach, he argues, wrote tropical medicine as 'a long, heroic history, commemorating the epochal movements through which the newly constituted specialty progressed from legend, mystery and medical geography in the eighteenth century to the organized colonial efforts of the 1880s. More recent historians, writes MacLeod, see it as a history which suggests that the distinction between tropical and temperate medicine is not so much one of the aetiology of disease as of politics and economics.[2] MacLeod argues that although different stages in the writing of the history of tropical medicine are apparent they have not been entirely progressive. The earlier approaches continue to be pursued by some historians, he argues, and publications in the last decade support this claim. The recent *Illustrated History of Tropical Diseases*, published by the Wellcome Trust, for instance, clearly adopts the early approach to the history of tropical medicine which seeks to document the 'discovery' of the diseases themselves and, more reasonably, the isolation of their causative agents and the discovery of cures and preventative measures. It is a fascinating book and an invaluable aid to the medical historian. It does, however, run the risk of leading the unwary into believing that the key factor in tropical medicine was, and remains, 'region' where region encompasses geography and, more importantly, race.[3] Its triumphalism also suggests that Western science alone had, and continues to have, the solution to the improved health of people living in the tropics. There is evidence, however, that in the medical world there has been a shift from viewing tropical medicine as a discipline with its nerve centre in the metropolis and its agents in tropical regions, to a view of 'medicine in the tropics'. Recent articles in *The Lancet*, *Medical Journal of Australia* and *Scottish Medical Journal* all acknowledge that while some diseases continue to have a devastating effect on populations living in the tropics and that other diseases are exclusive to tropical regions, it is cultural, economic and political issues that are profoundly important in establishing better health.[4]

Michael Worboys provides an excellent account of three recently published works on aspects of the history of tropical medicine. All three, with some limitations, could be placed in MacLeod's fourth phase in that they all clearly link economic and political situations to the health of the people and all make the point 'that tropical medicine was shaped by colonialism at every level'.[5] In her study of the influence of medical ideas and practice on the shaping of colonial images of Africa, Megan Vaughan is influenced by theories of social construction and seeks to elucidate cultural representations of disease. Of particular interest to this chapter is her discussion on the shaping of the 'Other' in defining and responding to disease within particular cultures. It is a point to which we will return when considering tropical medicine in Australia. The other two books reviewed by Worboys, John Farley's *Bilharizia* and Maryinez Lyons's *The Colonial Disease: A Social History of Sleeping Sickness in Northern Zaire* each focus, as their titles suggest, on a single disease. Farley uses Bilharzia as a case study to argue that tropical medicine was imperialist not only before the Second World War, an argument which he assumes will be widely accepted, but that it remained imperialist after the War, which he sees as a more contentious assertion.[6] Certainly, preliminary research in northern Australia would suggest that imperialistic health policies were pursued in post-war years.[7]

Similarly there are parallels between health policies applied to indigenous people in north Australia and those described by Lyons in her study of sleeping sickness in colonial Africa. But of particular interest here is Lyons' attempt to analyse the African response to the epidemic of sleeping sickness that affected Zaire in the early decades of the twentieth century. Her understanding of the African response was, she admits, constructed on white accounts of indigenous responses. An approach that relies on the extant records of colonists is limited in furthering any deeper understanding of African constructions of disease. It is useful, however, if recognised as a response visible to the coloniser and thus as understood and interpreted, and in turn responded to, by colonisers. While largely restricting herself to these parameters Lyons does, nevertheless, make greater claims for her analysis when she speculates on what an indigenous history of disease in this period might cover. She suggests that an African version of the history of the region would contain 'elements of truth' but does not elaborate on what 'untruths' it might also include.[8] Of importance here is the assumption that there is a 'true' history, rather than interpretations relevant to the position of the writer. My comments on Lyons' work, in fact, give undue emphasis to just one paragraph in a very comprehensive and detailed account of sleeping sickness. They are highlighted here in an effort to illustrate the limitations of writing about indigenous responses from which one might attempt to construct a picture of an indigenous identity. This is an important issue in this chapter. However, before this is explored further, a brief outline of tropical medicine in Australia will be useful.

In 1905 J. S. C. Elkington, one of Australia's noted public medical officers, produced a paper entitled 'Tropical Australia: Is it Suitable for a Working White Race?' It was presented first to a meeting of the Royal Society of Tasmania, and then published as a Commonwealth government paper.[9] It served to formally place on the government agenda an issue which had already received considerable public attention as both public servants and lay people alike had much to say on the subject, and it would remain a key medical issue in Australia in the following decades.

Tropical medicine as a distinct discipline in Australia arose from the intention of Australia's federal government to maintain the entire land mass of Australia for the nation. On federation in 1901, complete commitment had been given to a policy of 'white Australia'. An empty north – it would be over a half a century before the indigenous people would be counted as part of the Australian nation – was perceived as a threat to development of a white Australia. Should the teeming millions of Asia covet the Australian tropics, it would be difficult both morally and logistically to prevent their entry while it remained unoccupied. But the burning question, as indicated in the title of Elkington's paper, was, could a white race survive in the tropics? Elkington sidestepped the question of the economic worth of the tropical north in his paper, although this question in relation to the development of the north assumed greater importance in the following decades. Arguments about the economic potential of north Australia tended to run as a parallel debate to that of the health of the people as was illustrated in a cartoon published in the daily press when funding for tropical medical research was threatened during the depression of the 1930s.[10] In the cartoon politicians are being told that they must work hand-in-hand with the medical profession if they are intent upon establishing a white Australian community in the tropics. However, neither the economic nor the health question was seen to have been satisfactorily answered, and the Japanese threat, on the eve of the Second World War, dramatically changed the social, demographic, political and economic profile of northern Australia. And yet, for many years great faith had been placed in tropical medicine's power to assist with the development of northern Australia.

An Institute of Tropical Medicine, a Commonwealth government initiative, had been established at Townsville in northern Australia in 1911. Its primary purpose was:

> Firstly, the careful consideration of the question how far the insular isolation which Australia has enjoyed up to comparatively recent times with regard to disease will protect Australia in the future; secondly, the study of existing diseases in tropical Australia, and their prevention; thirdly, a thorough and impartial inquiry into the physiology of the

white race living and working under different conditions in tropical Australia.[11]

These three areas of activity, quarantine, endemic disease and physiological responses to the climate, became the defining characteristics of tropical medicine in Australia for as long as it survived as a distinct branch of medicine with dedicated facilities and separate funding.

It did not, however, survive long. By 1920, Anton Breinl, inaugural director of the Institute, was convinced that white people were as likely as any other to survive in the tropics; if he had not fully convinced all opponents they, at least, had no definitive evidence with which to contradict him. It was also apparent that only rarely had Australia suffered epidemic disease brought to its shores from Asia, or any other part of the world, and that established quarantine measures were a sufficient safeguard against such calamities. This left only endemic diseases. These, it was soon found, were not exclusively tropical. Indeed, many of the diseases found in the tropics were those also prevalent in the south. Thus, in a short space of time, the three imperatives of tropical medicine in Australia had been removed. In 1930 the Institute of Tropical Medicine was relocated in the south and merged with the School of Public Health at the University of Sydney. Despite failing to endure as a discipline, tropical medicine was not wholly without influence, and it did leave a legacy of formed attitudes and beliefs and a discourse about indigenous people and disease that was significant in the social and political history of northern Australia.

By 1911, when the Institute of Tropical Medicine was established in Australia, the six former colonies had been federated for a decade as the self-governing entity of the Commonwealth of Australia and to this extent Australia was no longer 'colonial'. In the north of Australia, however, colonialism continued. First, there was no seat of government in the north and tropical Australia continued to be administered from sites of extreme distance. In the Northern Territory the transfer of power from the South Australian to the Commonwealth government in 1911 had disenfranchised the entire population and those living in northern areas of Queensland and Western Australia were isolated from their governments by vast distances and limited transport and communication facilities.

Another element of a colonial world, a subject indigenous people, also survived. In Australia's southern populous areas, indigenous populations had been decimated as a result of settler expansion so that few identifiable groups remained. In the north, however, the indigenous population continued to be numerically superior, in the order of four to one for most of the period under discussion. Nor was there evidence to suggest that this large indigenous population could be successfully subjugated either physically or culturally. The vulnerability of the settler community was seen to lay at the point of contact with Aboriginal people. And it was here particularly that ideas of difference, couched only in negative terms, supported the adoption of the discourse of tropical medicine. The most common points of contact between settler and indigenous populations were sexual activity, domestic employment and schooling, all areas in which the imperatives of tropical medicine could be exercised.

These two factors alone were sufficient to engender the adoption of a particular identity by northern colonists. Other factors, however, such as the imperative of economic development and the perceived threat of invasion by other colonial powers, which will be discussed below, were also significant. For the colonial north of Australia the metropole was not Europe but the cities of settled Australia where economic survival was assured, a sense of nationalism was emerging and the indigenous population was so marginalised that it no longer impinged on the consciousness of the public or the policy-makers. In contrast, the north consisted of precariously situated settler communities uncertain of their survival, surrounded by vast tracts of unpatrolled and uncontrolled lands inhabited by indigenous people.

Tropical medicine in Australia has not yet been closely or comprehensively studied by historians, although some aspects of it have been discussed. In a comparative study of temperate medicine and settler capitalism Donald Denoon examines the racist nature of tropical medicine in Queensland and in Australia's mandated territory of Papua New Guinea.[12] Roy MacLeod and Donald Denoon's edited publication *Health and Healing in Tropical Australia and Papua New Guinea* contains some very well researched studies which would be useful to the historian who would make a comprehensive study of tropical medicine. My own detailed account of the role of health services in promoting white settlement in the Northern Territory could be used in this way. In this unpublished work I conclude that there was insufficient difference between the health problems encountered in northern Australia to sustain a distinction between tropical and temperate medicine but that nevertheless, racist imperatives of tropical medicine informed medical practice and policy formation.[13] Sufficient research to form the basis of a history of tropical medicine, except in the area of mission medicine, has now been completed but the focus of Australian historians in the last decade has largely turned to indigenous health with little consideration of tropical medicine, despite its importance, as part of that history.[14]

Although no comprehensive and detailed history has been written, broad parallels between tropical medicine in Australia and other colonial countries is already emerging. In his discussion of this aspect of history, Worboys suggests that the claim that tropical medicine rose to service the health needs of the colonisers is now familiar ground[15] and indeed, Denoon has already argued this in relation to Australia. Also familiar is the notion that the discourse of tropical medicine became a mechanism for the control of indigenous people in the interests of the colonisers and the way in which this happened in north Australia will be evident in the discussion below. It will, however, be the way in which such positioning shaped identity that will be the main focus here. It is not novel to suggest that responses to disease were framed in socially significant ways; as Charles Rosenberg reminds us, this is an ancient truth known by those who suffered disease in any historical period and social contructivist theories have lead us in this direction.[16] Further discussion of this point in respect of identity might, however, in light of some of the compelling claims made by indigenous Australians, serve to shed some light on contemporary health issues in Australia.

Indigenous and colonial identities

Claims made by Aboriginal people relate to both identity and to health and a response to them is needed before proceeding further. The first relates to identity and is well illustrated in the words of Aboriginal historian Jackie Huggins who writes:

> I detest the imposition that anyone who is non-Aboriginal can define my Aboriginality for me and my race. Neither do I accept any definition of Aboriginality by non-Aboriginals as it insults my intelligence, spirit and soul and negates my heritage. . . . There are no books written by non-Aboriginals that can tell them what it is to be Black as it is a fiction and an ethnocentric presumption to do so.[17]

Clearly, Huggins delineates the subject of indigenous identity as forbidden territory for non-Aboriginal historians. So, while to venture into the highly contested area of Aboriginal identity would be foolhardy, it must be considered here, as it will be argued that a shaping of the 'Other' was central to the formation of a colonial identity in northern Australia.

Further to this point, the grave difficulty of determining the extent to which colonial positioning of indigenous people was influential in the shaping of Aboriginal identity is acknowledged, particularly as historical records are silent on the subject. Available evidence stems almost exclusively from the written records of white males. Even where the voices of Aboriginal people are recorded they are filtered through the reporting procedures and conventions of colonial actors such as administrators, missionaries and doctors. The acceptance of oral history as a valid tool for gathering evidence has begun to allow greater exploration of indigenous history but is beyond the scope of this chapter. A recent conference on Aboriginal health, however, has made it abundantly evident that such issues cannot continue to be set aside as almost every Aboriginal speaker at that conference claimed that the continuing differential health problems of Aboriginal people in north Australia has it roots in a colonial past.[18] It will be surprising indeed to find that identities adopted by both the colonisers and the colonised were not a significant factor of that past.

The connection between identity and current health issues is the second issue raised by Aboriginal Australians. Before finally confining the discussion of indigenous identity to its counterpoint position in the construction of a northern colonial identity, a few observations can be made. In her work on the construction of an Australian indigenous identity, Deirdre Jordan argues that the construction of identity is not merely a question of self-identity. She argues that the location of the self by the self in society demands confirmation by others if a stable identity is to be realised. Jordan claims that 'for many Aborigines a syndrome of disturbance in identity formation has been caused by the process through which they have been identified' particularly where that identification 'has acted to nihilate the world of meaning of Aboriginal people, resulting in the location of their identity in negative characteristics'.[19] She cites several negative features of colonialism to support her argument and medical history may provide more.

One example drawn from medical history is the reaction of twenty Northern Territory Aboriginal women who were incarcerated in Darwin's quarantine station in 1937 when they were found to have contracted gonorrhoea. The Chief Medical Officer had demanded they, and another seven Aboriginal women, undergo medical examination when they were accused publicly of engaging in prostitution. The legitimacy of such an examination was doubtful in the regulations of the venereal disease legislation but could be effected under the provisions of the Aboriginal Ordinance. It was under the provisions of this ordinance also that the women were incarcerated for over 12 months. What is significant here is that several of the women, married with families, were exempt from the ordinance and could have challenged their isolation but did not do so. Could it be that they had been conditioned to compliance by their negative positioning? Nor was the selective and gendered application of the legislation challenged; Aboriginal women outside Darwin and Aboriginal men in or out of town were not isolated when infected with gonorrhoea. For white settlers and medical officials the compliance of the women confirmed the dangers of infectious diseases on the frontier. It also confirmed the need to adopt methods suited to frontier life. This is perhaps indicative of an acceptance of positioning within a colonial identity by at least one indigenous group but remains speculative in the absence of indigenous voices in extant historical records.

Another point on the subject of an indigenous identity which should be made relates to the multiplicity of positions taken by Aboriginal people in Australia. In the north this could be shaped by the nature of white incursion into Aboriginal lands, whether this was through pastoralism, missionary activities, bureaucratic control by police or medical officers, or the establishment of urban centres. Group and individual resolution of dilemmas were influenced by: the complexities of traditional law and the extent to which this had been maintained; access to traditional lands and freedom to use lands for traditional purposes; and the meaning attributed to social action whether within traditional boundaries and extending beyond them. To assume that there could be one indigenous identity would distort the complexity of relationships and, as Lynn Thomas argues in the context of African history, would flatten and distort the meaning-making of social action in a complex colonial environment.[20] There is some justification, however, for generalising about the negative positioning of Aboriginal people in the colonial context as being dangerous to the health of whites, as even those who saw merit in Aboriginal culture did not seek to redefine the image commonly portrayed of indigenous people. Rather, they demanded for them better levels of medical care. Typical of these is author Xavier Herbert who peoples his award-winning novel *Capricornia* and later, *Poor Fellow My Country*, with Aboriginal characters subject to the ravages of introduced diseases.

It has been suggested above that white identity was shaped in part through the positioning of indigenous people in particular ways. Closer examination will reveal the context and the complexities of white colonial identity in northern Australia. A level of generality will be employed here as there was an apparent wide acceptance of a group identity and a degree of compulsion to conform was exercised. For instance, in 1880 Dr Maurice was withdrawn from his position of Colonial Surgeon when he attempted to support several Aboriginal men accused of murdering two white miners. The social ostracism of pro-Aboriginal writer and government pharmacist Xavier Herbert in the 1930s is another case in point.[21] The unwillingness of some people to conform suggests that in some cases individual identity was stronger than group identity, although in the main there was a degree of compatibility between the two. Individual identity could, however, be impermanent. Many who came to the north in an official capacity came for a short, fixed period and so were able to adopt an alternative identity as a temporary measure. Such identities allowed considerable latitude as they could eventually be discarded in favour of one more suitable for inhabitants of the civilised south.

The question of cultural identity in the north of Australia has been explored by Jon Stratton. He argues that an identity which differs from Australia's metropolis has been both imposed on the north from the south, while at the same time a distinctive and separate identity is desired in the north. It is, he argues, an essential part of the Australian identity that Australians create the north as different and, in doing so, define themselves. If the north is tropical, impermanent, dangerous, a frontier, uncivilised and isolated, then Australians know the south to be temperate, permanent, safe, economically developed, civilised and central. The Northern Territory, writes Stratton, 'figures the limits of an Australian discursive system'.[22] Stratton argues that only now is the 'unsafe difference' of the past being made safe in the interests of the burgeoning tourist industry. But in the past, claiming difference and having difference acknowledged was an important part of identity in the colonial north. Being different, particularly where that difference encompassed the need to face danger and endure in an alien and inhospitable environment, carried its own rewards. Government officials in the north saw themselves as not having to conform to patterns of behaviour and bureaucratic processes established as being reasonable and acceptable in the south. When Paul Hasluck was appointed in the early 1950s as federal minister responsible for the Northern Territory with an unofficial mandate for welfare of all indigenous people, he claimed that the trouble with the people of the north was that they believed themselves to be different:

> this part of Australia was not thought of as a normal place to which normal practices and standards applied. . . . The Northern Territory was a place where things did not happen in the usual way and tasks were not done and life was not enjoyed in the same way as in the south.

He described the north as having a large population of old timers who were 'proudly isolationist and took grim satisfaction in being able to recall hardships' while the newcomers 'swaggered a little like intrepid characters who had put civilization behind them'. He found in the southern seat of government the north was 'regarded as a different and peculiar place'. He argued that such a position was false and counselled against the continuance of an attitude that condoned a relaxing of standards and allowed unorthodox, and even at times illegal, actions.[23] While it was widely accepted and argued that the north was different, there was no universal agreement on what that may constitute. Thus the shaping of difference could take a variety of forms. This is evident in the reaction of some medical men to the frequent writing of north Australia as a place where young men might succumb to venereal infection through sexual relations with indigenous women. They supported instead its difference being written in terms of a 'challenging frontier' that would attract 'spirited people' who would form the basis of a strong society in which a family could be raised.[24]

While in the south the 'Other' could be defined as the north, those in the north sought to position the indigenous population as all that the settler group was not. In his early and influential paper on whites in the tropics, however, Elkington had had very little to say about indigenous populations apart from the odd reference to 'coloured people' in other colonial settlements. Nor, when the Australian Institute of Tropical Medicine was established in 1910, did its charter make particular and specific reference to Aboriginal people, although they were implicitly implicated in the study of diseases endemic in the north. On the whole, the indigenous population was regarded as a problem, which would rapidly disappear as the north was settled and civilised, as had appeared to have been the case in the southern areas of Australia. Sir Raphael Cilento, Director of the Institute of Tropical Medicine from 1922 to 1930,[25] ascribed the early successful settlement of tropical Queensland to the absence of any 'teeming native coloured populations, riddled by endemic disease'.[26] It was an observation with which Anton Breinl agreed.[27] When Breinl was required by the Commonwealth government to make a health survey of the Northern Territory in 1911 he included those Aboriginal people living in close proximity to white settlement. He suggested a need to thoroughly research tropical diseases peculiar to Aboriginal people to ascertain their 'importance from the point of view of the settlement of the northern territory' but mentioned no immediate threat. However, foreshadowing what would become one of the most entrenched aspects of what might be called an Aboriginal health policy, he also suggested the need to ensure adequate control of disease amongst Aboriginal people through proper treatment. 'Like native races of other countries', he asserted, 'if a cure can be effected by one or two applications of a drug, the blackfellow is willing to undergo treatment; but should any prolonged treatment be necessary, then the aboriginal, with his childlike mind, does not persist, but soon evades further medication'.[28] So, from this early point, the discourse of tropical medicine included reference to an indigenous people entirely dependent on the settler population for a system of medical treatment well grounded in scientific methodology.

To dependency as a defining characteristic was added a particular conception of Aboriginal health. During the latter decades of the nineteenth century and the first two decades of the twentieth century the decline in the Aboriginal populations of Australia's tropical north had been rapid. It was repeatedly noted that Aboriginal people who had only minimal contact with white settlers and who continued to have ready access to their traditional food sources and land were able to maintain their good health.[29] Those in contact with whites, however, had been subject to serious epidemic and endemic disease. Major sites in which infection could occur were towns, but the mining and pastoral industries in which Aboriginal people found work were also a significant source of infection in the transmission of disease. It was repeatedly noted that Aboriginal people suffered high mortality rates through epidemics of measles, influenza and dysentery and when the influenza pandemic reached Darwin in 1919, Aboriginal mortality was reported to be high but, as the infection spread rapidly beyond the areas of white settlement, no estimate of overall mortality was recorded.[30]

Aboriginal groups also suffered badly from venereal diseases, malaria, leprosy and tuberculosis. Both syphilis and tuberculosis were reported to run a very swift course in Aboriginal patients, which lead to death in a matter of months rather than years. Both of these diseases were widespread in Aboriginal communities throughout northern Australia. In some Aboriginal groups the infection rate from venereal disease was reported to be as high as 90 per cent with children suffering to the same extent as their elders.[31] And, in the 1950s when the greatest damage had already been done, the exposure rate to tuberculosis in some groups was reported to be as high as 70 per cent.[32] Leprosy had become endemic in Aboriginal comminutes across the north, northeast and northwest coasts by the 1920s and during the 1930s many hundreds of Aboriginal people were isolated at the Channel Island Leprosarium in the Northern Territory and Peel and Fantome Islands in Queensland.[33] In the last malaria epidemic prior to the Second World War over two hundred Aboriginal people living near the Western Australian border died while other epidemics also resulted in high death rates.[34] Several attempts have been made to estimate Aboriginal depopulation following white settlement and studies of depopulation resulting from violence and from disease have been undertaken.[35] Similar studies for the Australian tropics are not yet available. From extant documentary evidence, however, the impact of disease introduced with white settlement can be judged to have been significant.

Thus, despite early conclusions that Australia's indigenous people had not been affected by introduced diseases to any large extent prior to colonisation, it was becoming increasingly evident that they were severely affected by diseases introduced through white settlement.[36] This of itself was not believed by the settler group to be a serious problem. It was, after all, inevitable that as the grand plan of Social Darwinism was played out the lesser races would succumb. To the coloniser the evidence was all too readily available. The difficulties Aboriginal people experienced in adopting new hygienic rules to suit the changed circumstances of their daily lives was plain to see. Sanitary measures in Aboriginal living areas on pastoral stations, mission stations and the less formally organised living areas on the fringes of towns were entirely inadequate. The adoption of different codes of dress without the accompanying hygienic measures led to a dramatic fall in health standards and could be directly related to the spread of specific diseases.[37] Inadequate nutrition also contributed to the failing health of Aboriginal people. Those most severely affected by these changing conditions were Aboriginal people living in close proximity to areas of white settlement. And, continuing the construction of settler-indigenous medical welfare established by Breinl, they were also the group most visible to settlers and the group most likely to come to the attention of medical officers. They became sites for the construction of the discourse as white settler opinions of Aboriginal health were shaped by observation of this section of the indigenous population. Whether Federal Aboriginal policy was segregation or, from 1939 on, assimilation, matters of hygiene would be of primary importance. Indeed, in the 1950s one of the principal aims of schooling for Aboriginal children was to teach hygiene. Paul Hasluck, the Commonwealth minister responsible for the Northern Territory in this period was to write, 'Aboriginal education is largely directed towards developing attitudes and personal habits, as well as knowledge, that will make aborigines socially acceptable to Europeans'.[38] Whereas in a framework of temperate medicine Aboriginal people might have been identified as individuals suffering ill-health, a positioning which would have evoked compassionate care and treatment, the discourse of tropical medicine identified them collectively as a diseased race and therefore a 'problem'.

Crucial in this defining of the 'Other' as diseased was the further positioning of indigenous people as not only unsupportive of northern development as that was seen by white settlers but as a direct threat to such development. 'Development', the goal of northern settlers, entailed the creation of an economic base though use of the land and was dependent on a healthy and vigorous white population. A diseased indigenous population was inimical to these aspirations and there crept into the discourse references to them as threatening the health of the white settler population. Threats to the health of the settler population would stem first, he and others argued, from a lack of hygiene in Aboriginal living areas and, secondly, from Aboriginal susceptibility to introduced disease. Aboriginal groups would, it was argued, become a constant source of infection for the white population. Such had been the experience in other colonial settings and thus it also became part of the discourse of tropical medicine in Australia and continues today. It is, for instance, a reoccurring theme in the public debate on the spread of HIV infection and centres around concerns of it entering the Aboriginal population.

In 1931 Cilento presented a report to the Federal Health Council of Australia in which he warned that in the Aboriginal population there was an untouched field of granuloma and yaws and that there could be no doubt that the Aboriginal people 'represent a foci for the dissemination of hookworm, malaria, and other diseases'.[39] In the same report Cilento presented a map to illustrate the need for continued vigilance in quarantine given the close proximity of tropical Australia to Asian and Pacific nations and the potential for introduced disease to affect an unimmunised and highly susceptible indigenous population. A few years later he reported that the incidence of leprosy in Queensland corresponded 'very roughly with the degree of prevalence of coloured persons in the population'.[40] Cook, in his first major policy statement following his appointment as Chief Medical Officer, argued that maintaining a white Australia in the north would be complicated by

> the preponderating aboriginal. The aboriginal has no system of medicine or practical sanitation in his civilisation. It is incumbent on the white race directly or indirectly responsible for the introduction of so many factors of morbidity and mortality to make good this deficiency in the interests of both races . . . The prevalence of Malaria and Venereal diseases in aboriginals is a perennial menace to the white settler. Contact between aboriginals and foreign carriers of diseases must be controlled to prevent dissemination by the migration of the former.[41]

Few administrators would be as outspoken as Cook regarding the Aboriginal threats to white health. More commonly, such concerns were hidden beneath a paternalistic solicitude for Aboriginal health. As Tim Rowse has observed in relation to rationing, the paternalistic morality of the settler group allowed the preeminence of a discourse other than that of indigenous rights,[42] and while a system of health 'care' was imposed on the indigenous population, moral concerns could be said to have been observed. Whatever the stated reason, however, the resulting action was similar. The entrenched racism of this period of Australian history, which was grounded in Social Darwinism and eugenic theories, is now well known and has received considerable attention from historians. It need not be repeated here, but it is useful to observe that the discourse of tropical medicine where it involved Australia's indigenous people was consistent with attitudes at the time and significantly provided what was seen as scientific support for them.

During this period, the identification of a problem carried with it the belief that a scientific approach would bring about a solution. In his seminal work on bourgeois social thought and 'progressivism' in Australia, Michael Roe notes that a belief in both science and scientific methods reached its height in the first half of the twentieth century. The confidence of the progressivist was in efficiency gained through scientific investigation and effective action pursued by bureaucratic and other élites.[43] Figuring prominently amongst Australia's progressivists was Elkington and J. H. L. Cumpston, appointed federal Director General of Health in 1921, a position that made him particularly influential in issues of tropical medicine. Other leading medical men were also convinced of the value of science and were imbued with a sense of duty, which included a duty to protect northern settlers from disease through the scientific application of rapidly expanding medical knowledge. For some the sense of duty extended to indigenous people, leading one medical officer to report in that 1917 Aboriginal people confined in the town compound for medical treatment were grateful for relief from distressing and painful conditions.[44] It was missionaries, however, who were more likely to encompass within their duty to Aboriginal people the provision of modern scientific medical assistance. The perplexity and occasional indignation of missionaries when either their ministrations were not gratefully received, or introduced scientific approaches not adopted, is evident. Clearly, professional and lay faith in scientific solutions to the problems of tropical medicine and the 'problem' of Aboriginal people were great.

Responses to a colonial identity

Given the goal of those in the north to lay claims to the land in the interests of the nation, and the physical dangers to be faced in pursuit of this goal, what then was the response? Both responding to, and shaping, a northern identity was the position taken by Cecil Cook. When applying for the position of Chief Medical Officer of the Northern Territory in 1927, he argued that there was no way that he could adequately attend to the health of whites without having full control of the Aboriginal population. Consequently, he was appointed not only to the most senior medical position but also to the position of Chief Protector of Aborigines. In the Northern Territory and the north of Western Australia medical concerns provided a major reason for the control of Aboriginal people and official intervention in Aboriginal lives until very recent times was more likely to be for medical than any other reason. In Queensland it became another justification for a system of control through reserves.[45] The historian Mary Anne Jebb has argued that the spread of venereal disease amongst Aboriginal people in the northern areas of

Western Australia, and the threat it posed to both the white settlers and the black labour force on which the pastoral industry depended, resulted in 1905 in the promulgation of an Aborigines Act.[46] The policy enshrined in the legislation was the segregation of Aboriginal people, the most immediate and dramatic results of which will be discussed below. Legislation for the Northern Territory was couched in terms of the protection of Aboriginal people and gave to the Chief Protector of Aborigines responsibility for the 'supply of food, medical attendance, medicines and shelter for the sick, aged and infirm aboriginals'. More importantly, or at least, made more important by administrators and public officials, was another section of the ordinance which allowed the Chief Protector to remove any Aboriginal person to a designated Aboriginal institution or reserve.[47] When linked, these two sections of the Ordinance allowed the Chief Protector to remove Aboriginal people to institutions for health reasons and a number of detention facilities such as the Channel Island Leprosarium were registered as Aboriginal institutions for the purpose of this Ordinance. In Queensland, rigidly enforced segregation on reserves were established under the 1897 Aborigines Protection and Restriction of the Sale of Opium Act, legislation which, Ray Evans argues, was prompted both by humanitarian concerns and an effort to save the sensibilities of whites from the sight of fringe dwelling Aboriginal people living in extremes of poverty and disease.[48] In Queensland it was later administrators, such as Cilento, who took advantage of the already established reserve system to support principles of tropical medicine.

In some cases, legislation relating to specific diseases was also introduced in addition to established public health acts. In all states leprosy was listed as an infectious disease in general health legislation but in Queensland a separate Leprosy Act was passed in 1892. Leprosy had been introduced into late nineteenth-century Queensland with labour imported from the Pacific islands and with Chinese immigration but it was the spread of the disease amongst the Aboriginal population which caused the greatest alarm. Some decades later this epidemiological pattern was replicated in the Northern Territory and the Ordinance for the Suppression of Leprosy was introduced in 1928. I have argued elsewhere that the isolation of leprosy patients on island institutions, which stemmed from this legislation, was maintained, long after comparable institutions in other countries had been moved to mainland centres, as a direct response to the majority of patients being Aboriginal.[49]

Legislation relating to venereal diseases, promulgated in the nineteenth century under public health or infectious diseases acts and in specific legislation at the time of the First World War,[50] cannot be understood in terms of race alone as gender and class[51] were powerful factors in their introduction, but in northern Australia attitudes to race allowed the introduction of even greater discrimination. When introduced in the Northern Territory in 1923 the Venereal Disease Ordinance was in line with that introduced in other parts of Australia and was mainly concerned with notification. Changes introduced in 1933 dictated the time, place and length of treatment and established a register of infected persons. In the Northern Territory lock hospitals for Aboriginal patients suffering from venereal disease were, from time to time, established under the Aboriginals Ordinance as they were not sanctioned under health laws. In 1937 Cook gained the support, albeit reluctant support, of the Commonwealth Director-General of Health for changes to the Venereal Disease Ordinance, 1928, which, had administrative changes not prevented it being enacted, would have allowed medical officers to compulsorily examine not only those 'reasonably suspected' of having venereal disease but all 'coloured' people who escaped the net of the Aboriginal Ordinance. In Western Australia the lock hospitals on two barren islands off the north-west coast, which operated between 1908 and 1919, were also established under legislation relating to Aboriginal people. Similarly, in Queensland Aboriginal ordinances were used to isolate those suffering venereal disease on Fantome Island or in lock hospitals. A 1934 amendment to the Act gave protectors power to examine any Aboriginal person suspected of having venereal disease. Cilento too targeted the 'crossbreed and alien coloured elements' who were not subject to the Aboriginal Protection Act as agents in the spread of 'disease and vice'.[52]

During periods when white settlement was sparse, the banishment of Aboriginal people from settled areas was common and, as the land was increasingly occupied by white settlers, there was a corresponding increase in the use of segregation supported by protectionist legislation. Ray Evans has documented a persistent recourse in Queensland's colonial period to the banishment of Aboriginal people in the face of an infectious epidemic or widespread infection with venereal disease, leprosy or tuberculosis.[53] He cites the Aboriginal protector for the Urandangie area who, when faced with an influenza epidemic amongst local Aboriginal people in 1900, wrote:

> [My] informants feared an Epidemic might break out among the white children in the town and suggested that the blacks should be isolated . . . I ordered them to be removed to a waterhole one mile from the town. . . . This is all that can be done for them at the present.

Similarly, early cases of leprosy found in the Northern Territory were removed from the town and sent back to their traditional lands, a policy which was still being advocated in 1906 by Ramsay Smith, the senior South Australian Public Health Official. Ramsay Smith recommended banishment rather than isolation in the belief that 'in the Northern Territory one is not dealing with an overcrowded, or even crowded, population of whites – among whom the blacks may spread leprosy'.[54] In 1925 the District Medical Officer at Derby in Western Australia's north speculated that that the increasingly high disease amongst Aboriginal people living in remote areas was due to the practice of 'sending natives "bush" when sick to avoid the expenses of treatment'.[55] When, as happened on several occasions, ships arrived in Darwin harbour carrying Chinese immigrants suffering from smallpox, all Aboriginal people were ordered out of town. In the face of the influenza pandemic following the First World War, it was planned that all Aboriginal people would be moved to the other side of the harbour if the infection gained entry to the town. In the event, torrential Wet Season rains prevented the move and as an alternative measure, all Aboriginal people living in the vicinity of the town were confined to the town reserve. There, in overcrowded conditions, the infection spread rapidly. In both Western Australia and the Northern Territory a line of latitude delineating tropical and non-tropical Australia, over which Aboriginal people were forbidden to cross in north or south travel, was declared for the control of leprosy and poliomyelitis, respectively.[56]

Aboriginal people could be subjected to compulsory medical examination and, in northern pastoral regions, the 'raiding' of Aboriginal living areas by police officers for the purpose of enforced medical examinations was common practice. Repeatedly, such practices were justified in terms of the protection of the settler community, with those elements of the discourse of tropical medicine outlined above being drawn upon. As late as 1949 Cook was still claiming that:

> The pernicious influences which the coloured races exercise upon the hygienic, social and economic development of areas where white settlement is sparse, and upon public health where hybrid remnants concentrate in the poorer quarters of cities or on the fringes of towns, continues for the most part unsuspected.[57]

By this time, however, while concern continued to be expressed about the standards of hygiene amongst Aboriginal groups, isolation and segregation were no longer favoured as matters of policy.

Whether as a result of legislation relating specifically to Aboriginal people or that enacted for the governance of the entire population, Aboriginal people were controlled as a measure against the spread of infection. Compulsory segregation and restrictions on movements were not confined to tropical Australia, as indicated by the exclusion of Aboriginal children from schools[58] and general bans on Aboriginal people entering country towns except for the purposes of work.[59] The discourse of tropical medicine, however, added to the legitimacy of such policies through the provision of a scientific rationale. It was the discourse of difference in the shaping of identity that legitimised and continued to sanction the imperatives of tropical medicine.

As noted earlier, Deirdre Jordan has argued that the construction of identity requires a level of confirmation by others. A northern identity defined itself in terms of its struggle to establish a white settlement in an alien and threatening environment that called for the exercise of power over an indigenous people. But, to what extent was this reflected by those living in southern, temperate Australia? Clearly, Paul Hasluck did little to confirm such self-identification but he was influential only at the end of the period in question. There was, however, extensive support for seeing the north of Australia as different. Unpopulated, it remained a threat to real Australia with fears of an Asian invasion seen in policies to combat the 'yellow peril'.[60] Those who would take on the task of maintaining the north in the best interests of the nation would be men of strength and independence who would, ideally, be supported by resourceful, hard-working women.

There was too apparent confirmation from those defined as the 'Other'. Suggestive of this was the continuing decline in Aboriginal health, which has not yet been overcome. Today, there are consistent calls for Aboriginal people to take greater responsibility for their own health,[61] and there is evidence that this apparent lack of involvement with health care was a response shaped in colonial times. Segregation and isolation by colonisers as a response to ill health was the common experience of Aboriginal people and the resulting fear and loss of liberty are living memories in Aboriginal communities. Such positioning left Aboriginal people with little power when dealing with ill health. This is not to suggest, however, that there was an universal acceptance of an imposed positioning. Aboriginal people consistently resisted medical attention that might result in their removal from country and 'escapes' from places of confinement were common. This served to reinforce for the colonisers the danger of their position and confirm their need for strength and vigilance.

If indeed the negative position of Aboriginal people in terms of health and hygiene has influenced an indigenous self-identity, then there is ample evidence that this is being reshaped today. One of the most powerful movements in indigenous health in the last decade has been the demand that control of health resources to be entrusted to indigenous organisations. The result has been a burgeoning of health services run by indigenous people for indigenous people. Indicative of the re-assertion of cultural identity in the wake of the assimilation policy and its connection with health issues is the 'Strong Women, Strong Babies, Strong Culture' programme. Here, indigenous health workers seek to re-assert a cultural identity that is positive and gives women control over their bodies. They write: 'If the traditional structures of Aboriginal life are strong, and we are building new ways into our life then we will be able to overcome all of the conflicts and problems. We will have the right prevention and protection'.[62] Although now, at least in policy, negative positioning of Aboriginal people has been avoided, a positive cultural acceptance has not been fully incorporated. The delivery of medical and health services remains deeply embedded in Western cultural understandings.

If Aboriginal culture is still largely overlooked, policies of self-determination for Aboriginal people have reintroduced cultural considerations, at least where the channels for funding are being negotiated. Some funds for medical programmes are now being distributed through the agency of the Aboriginal and Torres Strait Islander Commission and the whole area of funds for medical services to the Aboriginal community is now hotly contested.[63] There is, however, obvious concern in some quarters that cultural issues are not being given sufficient consideration in the planning and execution of medical programmes, a deficiency which is contributing to the on-going poor health of Aboriginal groups in Australia. Now, at a time when so-called 'life-style' diseases rather that infectious diseases pose the greatest threat to Aboriginal health, it is imperative that culture be taken into consideration in developing medical programmes. At the risk of stating the obvious, and certainly restating what numerous others have said, improvement in Aboriginal health will not happen in isolation from improved living conditions for Aboriginal people and their greater autonomy within Australian society. Identity remains an issue of great importance.

While the discourse of tropical medicine in the shaping of identity has been explored here largely in terms of race with important intersections with gender, gender and sexuality still require further investigation in which the importance of masculinity in shaping identity on Australia's frontier can be more fully explored.[64] Nevertheless, it can be argued that in northern Australia white settlers constructed an identity that distinguished itself from that of southern, settled Australia and clearly positioned itself in spatial and racial terms. Further, it can be argued that tropical conditions, including notions of tropical medicine, contributed to that identity. The positioning of indigenous people in relation to a Western scientific paradigm is not locked away in colonial times; it can be seen in current medical practice. Understanding the ways in which it operates is crucial to moving on from a colonial past.

Notes

1 Geoffrey Stokes, 1997, *The Politics of Identity in Australia*, Cambridge University Press, Melbourne.
2 R. MacLeod and M. Lewis, 1988, *Disease, Medicine and Empire: Perspectives on Western Medicine and the Experience of European Expansion*, Routledge, London, pp. 4–6.
3 See for example reference to the people of Papua New Guinea as 'stoneage', F. E. G. Cox (ed.), 1996, *Illustrated History of Tropical Medicine*, The Wellcome Trust, London, p. 154.
4 B. Currie, 1993, 'Medicine in Tropical Australia', *Medical Journal of Australia*, Vol. 158, 3 May, pp. 609–15; Editorial, 1996, 'Will Tropical Medicine Move to the Tropics?', *The Lancet*, Vol. 347, No. 9002, p. 629; G. C. Cook, 1993, 'Tropical Medicine: A Changing Scenario', *Scottish Medical Journal*, Vol. 38, No. 1, pp. 7–11.
5 M. Worboys, 1995, Book Review, *Social History of Medicine*, Vol. 8, No. 2, pp. 331–4.
6 J. Farley, 1991, *Bilharzia: A History of Imperial Tropical Medicine*, Cambridge University Press, Cambridge, pp. 3–4.
7 See for instance Julie Wells, 1995, 'The Long March: Assimilation Policy and Practice in Darwin the Northern Territory, 1939–1967', PhD Thesis, University of Queensland.

8. Maryinez Lyons, 1992, *The Colonial Disease: a Social History of Sleeping Sickness in Northern Zaire, 1900–1940*, Cambridge University Press, Cambridge, p. 167.
9. J. S. C. Elkington, 1905, 'Tropical Australia: Is it Suitable for a Working White Race?' Commonwealth Parliamentary Paper.
10. *Daily Mail*, 28 July 1933.
11. Anton Breinl, 1913, 'The Object and Scope of Tropical Medicine in Australia', *Australasian Medical Congress Transactions*, Vol. 1, p. 526.
12. D. Denoon, 1988, 'Temperate Medicine and Settler Capitalism', in R. MacLeod and M. Lewis (eds), *Disease, Medicine and Empire*, pp. 119–20.
13. Suzanne Parry, 1992, 'Disease, Medicine and Settlement', PhD Thesis, University of Queensland.
14. For example see Ernest Hunter, 1993, *Aboriginal Health and History*, Cambridge University Press, Melbourne.
15. Worboys, 1995, Book Review, p. 331.
16. Charles Rosenberg, 1992, 'Framing Disease: Illness, Society and History', in Charles Rosenberg and Janet Golden (eds), *Framing Disease: Studies in Cultural History*, Rutgers University Press, New Jersey.
17. Jackie Huggins, 1993, 'Always was always will be', *Australian Historical Studies*, No. 100, April, p. 459.
18. See Gary Robertson, 1996, *Aboriginal Health: Social and Cultural Transitions*, NT University Press, Darwin.
19. Deirdre Jordan, 1985, 'Census Categories – Enumeration of Aboriginal People, or Construction of Identity?', *Australian Aboriginal Studies*, No. 1, p. 29.
20. Cited in Nancy Rose Hunt, 1996, 'Introduction', *Gender and History*, Vol. 8, No. 3, p. 326.
21. See Suzanne Saunders, 1990, 'Another Dimension: Xavier Herbert in the Northern Territory', *Journal of Australian Studies*, No. 26, pp. 52–65.
22. Jon Stratton, 1989, 'Reconstructing the Territory', *Cultural Studies*, Vol. 3, No. 1, p. 54.
23. Paul Hasluck, *Shades of Darkness: Aboriginal Affairs, 1925–1965*, Melbourne University Press, Melbourne, p. 82–3.
24. See comments of J. T. Beckett recorded in Report of the Administrator, 1914.
25. For detailed discussion of Cilento see A. T. Yarwood, 1991, 'Sir Raphael Cilento and the White Man in the Tropics', in Roy MacLeod and Donald Denoon, *Health and Healing in Tropical Australia and Papua New Guinea*, James Cook University, Townsville.
26. Raphael Cilento, 1923, 'Australia's Special Problems in Tropical Hygiene', *Health*, Vol. 1, No. 2, p. 39.
27. Anton Breinl, 1920, 'Figures and Facts Regarding Health and Disease in Northern Australia Influencing Its Permanent Settlement by a White Race', *Transactions of the Australian Medical Congress*.
28. Anton Breinl, 1912, 'Report on Health and Disease in the Northern Territory', in *Report of Preliminary Scientific Expedition to the Northern Territory*, Australian Commonwealth Government, Melbourne, pp. 52–3.
29. Report of the Administrator, Northern Territory of Australia, 1913–17.
30. Ibid., 1920, p. 62.
31. Raymond Evans, 1975, 'The Condition of the Aboriginal Remnant', in Raymond Evans, Kay Saunders and Kathy Cronin (eds), *Exclusion, Exploitation and Extermination: Race Relations in Colonial Queensland*, Australia and New Zealand Book Company, Sydney, pp. 85–101.
32. Australian Archives Canberra (AAC), A431, 49/422.
33. See Suzanne Saunders, 1986, '"A Suitable Island Site": Leprosy in the Northern

Territory and the Channel Island Leprosarium', BA(Hons) Thesis, Murdoch University.
34 Edward Ford, 1950, 'The Malaria Problem in Australian and the Australian Pacific Territories', *Medical Journal of Australia*, Vol. 1, No. 23, pp. 749–60.
35 For example see Henry Reynolds, 1981, *The Other Side of the Frontier*, History Department, James Cook University, Townsville; Noel Butlin, 1983, *Our Original Aggression*, George Allen and Unwin, Sydney.
36 For one example see Australian Archives Northern Territory (AANT), A3, 22/2805, Medical Report by Herbert Basedow.
37 For details see Suzanne Parry, 1992, 'Disease, Medicine and Settlement: the Role of Health and Medical Services in the Settlement of the Northern Territory', PhD Thesis, University of Queensland, ch. 4.
38 AAC, A1361/1, 45/3/1, Part 6.
39 Raphael Cilento, 1931, 'Review of the Position of Tropical Medicine and Hygiene in Australia', Report of the Federal Health Council, 5th Session.
40 R. W. Cilento, 1934, 'Brief Review of Leprosy in Australia and Its Dependencies', *Proceedings of the Federal Health Council*, 7th Session.
41 AAC, A1928/1, 362/11.
42 Tim Rowse, 1999, 'Rationing's Moral Economy', in T. Austin and S. Parry (eds), *Connection and Disconnection*, Northern Territory University Press, Darwin.
43 Michael Roe, 1984, *Nine Australian Progessives: Vitalism in Bourgeois Social Thought, 1890–1960*, University of Queensland Press, St Lucia, p. 11
44 Report of the Administrator, Northern Territory, 1917, p. 37.
45 See Noel Loos, 1993, 'A Chapter of Contact: Aboriginal–Europeans Relations in North Queensland, 1606–1992', in Henry Reynolds, *Race Relations in North Queensland*, James Cook University, Townsville.
46 Mary Anne Jebb, 1987, 'Isolating the Problem: Venereal Disease and Aborigines in Western Australia, 1898–1924', BA(Hons) Thesis, Murdoch University.
47 Northern Territory Aboriginals Ordinance, 1912, Section 16(1).
48 Ray Evans, 1975, 'Epilogue: The Last Round-up', in Ray Evans, Kay Sanders and Kathy Cronin, 1975, *Exclusion, Exploitation and Extermination*, p. 119.
49 Suzanne Saunders, 1990, 'Leprosy Prophylaxis in Australia', *Aboriginal History*, Vol. 14, pp. 168–81.
50 J. H. L. Cumpston, 1920, 'Venereal Disease in Australia: Report of the Royal Commission on Health', Commonwealth Government Printer.
51 See Kay Daniels (ed.), 1984, *So Much Hard Work: Women and Prostitution in Australian History*, Fontana Collins, Sydney.
52 Quoted in Milton Lewis, 1998, *Thorns on the Rose: the History of Sexually Transmitted Diseases in Australia in International Perspective*, AGPS Press, Canberra.
53 Ray Evans, 1975, 'The Condition of the Remnant', in Ray Evans *et al.*, *Exclusion, Exploitation and Extermination*, pp. 98–101.
54 W. Ramsay Smith, 1906, 'Hygiene in the Northern Territory', South Australian Government, Adelaide.
55 Quoted in W. S. Davidson, 1978, *Havens of Refuge*, University of Western Australia Press, Perth, p. 166.
56 Suzanne Parry, 1992, 'Disease, Medicine and Settlement', p. 314; W. A. Davidson, 1978, *Havens of Refuge*.
57 C. E. Cook, 1949, 'The Native in Relation to the Public Health', *Medical Journal of Australia*, 30 April, p. 569.
58 J. J. Fletcher, 1989, *Clean, Clad and Courteous: A History of Aboriginal Education in New South Wales*, J. Fletcher, Carlton.
59 Anna Haebich, 1992, *For their Own Good: Aborigines and the Government in*

the South West of Western Australia, 1900–1940, University of Western Australia Press, Perth.
60 See Alan Powell, 1996, *Far Country: A Short History of the Northern Territory*, Melbourne University Press, Melbourne.
61 See for instance statements made by the Chief Minister to the Foreign Correspondents' Association of Australia, 6 July 1993.
62 Lorna Fejo and Cheryl Rae, 1996, 'Strong Women, Strong Babies, Strong Culture Project', in Gary Robinson, *Aboriginal Health*, p. 81.
63 Michael Hall, 1994, 'Politics of Aboriginal Health in the Northern Territory', BA(Hons) Thesis, Northern Territory University.
64 For examples elsewhere see Robert MacDonald, 1993, *Sons of the Empire: the Frontier and the Boy Scout Movement, 1890–1918*, University of Toronto Press, Toronto.

7 Colonial doctors and national myths
On telling lives in Australian medical biography*

Roy Macleod

Introduction

'Biography,' Philip Guedalla once said, 'is a very definite region, bounded on the north by history, on the south by fiction, on the east by obituary notices, and on the west by tedium.'[1] To which it may be appropriate to apply the motto of Sydney University: sidere mens eadem mutato (the same spirit under the southern skies). Biography is today big business, north and south. The Library of Congress reports that through the 1980s, biography was (at 15 per cent) the most popular category of non-fiction in the US, rivalling action and historical novels.

In Australia, biography vies with autobiography for a place in the invention of national identity. Jill Ker Conway, Bernard Smith, Donald Horne are modern instalments of a genre that dates from Miles Franklin, Henry Handel Richardson, and Christina Stead. The craft was not always promising. In the 1890s, Henry Lawson's advice to 'any Australian writer whose talents have been recognised,' was 'to go steerage; stow away, swim and seek London, Yankeeland or Timbuctoo – rather than stay in Australia, till his genius turned to gall or beer. Or, failing this, to study elementary anatomy ... and then shoot himself carefully.'[2] Fortunately, at least some of the European medical practitioners who came to Australia knew elementary anatomy, and did not shoot themselves – and left us stories and telling lives.

Within the last five years, there has been a growing interest in writing lives of the medical men and women who, for a time at least, have called Australia home. Library searches reveal a seven-fold jump in biographical articles between 1970 and 1989 – from 5 to 36 – and a steady increase during the 1990s, of about 5 per year. At the same time, however, there has been little scholarly study of the phenomenon of medical biography, and even less of the images of an imagined past it imparts to the present. This may be contrasted with the history of science in Australia, which over the last fifteen years has seen over 1,100 biographical references, of which 538 are new to scholarship.[3] Moreover, changing fashions and tendencies in science life-writing have been canvassed repeatedly by conferences at Toronto in 1980, London in 1987, Sydney in 1988, Hamburg in 1989, Canberra in 1992, and

London again in 1994. For reasons we may wish to explore, the study of medical biography remains in its infancy. And within that, colonial medical biography has hardly begun.

My question is: why? In an era in which there have been such rich harvests awaiting the biographically inclined, and such popular interest – why have there been so few professional takers? And why so little academic recognition? The answers, I suggest, are instructive, and lie beyond the business of writing books – although not perhaps the business of selling them. In Australia, as elsewhere, the search for an answer may tell us much about the ways in which a people have viewed themselves and wish others to view them.

Some of the obstacles confronting colonial medical biography are clear enough. Whilst biographers in the Newton, Darwin, Einstein, and Freud industries have established a place for what is 'human' in the history of science – as long as Blackwells find they can make money in 'Science Biographies',[4] and whilst of biographical dictionaries of scientists, there seems to be no end[5] – medical biography has found little enthusiasm among Australian publishers. The fourteen bibliographies of the history of Australian science produced by Laurie Carlson of Deakin University since 1980, list twenty colonial biographies as appearing during the last twenty-five years. But of these, fewer than half have been produced by Australian publishers. Therein lies a second conundrum. If science biography is fundamentally about ideas and success, medical biography is about people and situations. If science biography likes its heroes to be revolutionaries, and gives prizes to those who win, medical biography tolerates failures. For medical history, it is the journey as much as the arrival that commands attention. That journey inevitably explores new boundaries. To comprehend the person, the practitioner, and the place requires a particular blend of professional skills.

This combination is particularly unusual in the once-colonial world, where the organised study of medical history is still in its adolescence. Today, there are 400 members of the Australian Society for the History of Medicine, of whom only 10 are professionals. The subject is far from industrial sed, or even specialised, and is proudly an amateur avocation, dominated by heroic narratives of bush medicine and base hospitals, and narratives of distinguished figures in tropical public health, nursing, and health administration. In this context, medical biography is a cinderella speciality, living somewhere between family history and the fraternal obituary, and has yet to establish standards. Indeed, its practice – and its practitioners – have exposed themselves to the same criticisms that Lytton Strachey aimed at his Eminent Victorians, except that fewer may be eminent, and by no means all are Victorians.

If few medical historians would dismiss biography, but few pause to consider it as a genre, fewer still are interested in how it fares when it travels to the outposts of the colonial periphery. The fact is that the colonial medical profession in Australia – that is, before Federation, but possibly also until the 1930s, when it was still shaped by colonial attitudes and institutions – was not always heroic, nor particularly noble in the annals of diagnosis, or clinical procedure – nor until the generation of Macfarlane Burnett and the Eliza and Walter Hall Institute was it noted for its outstanding contributions to new knowledge. That it has become so today, is a proud story of contemporary Australia, about which much can be said.

Two hundred years ago, however, our present past was a distinctly foreign country. European biography in Australia began with European settlement – and in a formal sense, enjoyed, or endured, characteristics similar to those found throughout in the English-speaking world. But from its penal origins, life in the austral Eden acquired a special complexion – as convicts and traders, soldiers and settlers, lawyers and doctors wrested their identity uncertainly from a British willingness to let go, and from the grip of distance, drought, and desert that refused to engage.[6] Biography had to force its way against a mainstream tradition dominated by what Geoffrey Blainey has called a 'black-arm band' vision of history, in which the profession, closely allied to the police power, were viewed with cynicism and distrust; and where the ethos of service was held at a discount. The land and its people shaped medical practice. But the human and physical obstacles of nature with which medicine had to contend were almost insuperable. 'In all directions,' one of Patrick White's characters recalls,

> stretched the Great Australian Emptiness in which the mind is the least of possessions, in which the rich man is the important man, in which the schoolmaster and the journalist rule what intellectual roost there is, in which beautiful youths and girls stare at life through blind blue eyes, in which human teeth fall like autumn leaves, the buttocks of cars grow hourly glassier, food means cake and steak, and the march of material ugliness does not raise a quiver from the average nerves.[7]

John Rickard has suggested that biography in Australia has not until recently been a subject of methodological concern, because it 'hitched a ride on the coat tails of history', and rested content within broad, essential outlines, rather than 'in human terms, explaining the person concerned'.[8] It was almost impossible, the argument runs, to engage with the medical geographies of the great south land, its unfamiliar insects and plants, its paradoxical animals – the 'land of contrarieties', as Darwin put it – given the white man's haunting ignorance of a fathomless Aboriginal dreamtime, encircled like a symbolic snake by its own deep resonance with nature.

Such reasons may help to explain why medical biography in Australia has yet to find its Michael Holroyds, or even its Peter Careys. James Walter has suggested that 'the post-colonial cultural space is still not one conductive to theories of the self'.[9] For colonised Australia and New Zealand, the definitional 'other' has been the coloniser, who has defined the questions and set the agenda. Until the late 1960s, when the *Australian Dictionary of Biography* – the *ADB* – began, Australian biographers despaired of their task – in Manning Clark's phrase, 'so pitifully afraid of the light'.[10] The burden of colonial stereotypes was suffocating; and secondary sources were biased by an imperial perspective.

However, in the last decade, 'fear' has given way to confidence, and to the assertion of primacy in identity and place. A biographical culture is emerging in which creativity is commemorated in context, and in which local and characteristic modes of thought appear the more valuable for being shaped by local conditions, rather than by enlightening rays emanating from the metropolis. Certainly, the writing of *colonial* biography is assuming a role in national *self*-biography, and in this, colonial *medical* biography occupies a significant place. In the determination of the Australian biographical 'self', the *ADB* has played a path-breaking part.

The *ADB* and colonial medics

In announcing its revisionist charter the *New Dictionary of National Biography* – the *New DNB* – now being published by Oxford University Press, has indicated its interest in including more colonial entries, and to revise those it already has. Through its editorial brief runs the suggestion that earlier biographies have reinforced dated stereotypes, without signalling significant changes.

The same concern runs through a close reading of the *ADB*, established in 1957, as a joint venture between Australian National University and the Melbourne University Press, and since the flagship of Australian biographical nationalism. Strachey once sneered at what he called 'undertakers', whose three-deckered 'Lives and Letters' left scholars such a rich resource. Australia has had no such tradition. Instead, it has the *ADB*, egalitarian and austere, attempting to combine honesty with charity, in sparing prose. Its formulae owe much to the example of Strachey's *DNB*, and to a lesser extent, the *Dictionary of American Biography* – and so it records the 'cv's' of the famous, the near famous, and the interesting.

But then it begins to differ. Entries are proposed by ordinary citizens, vetted by state committees, and after consultation, selected by the editorial staff in Canberra. Over its forty years, it has followed the 'floruit' principle, with thirteen volumes devoted to four periods – (1) 1780–1850, (2) 1851–1890, (3) 1891–1939, and (4) those who died between 1940–1980.[11] Figures in science, engineering and medicine comprise about 10 per cent of the entries – 800 of the total of 7,891 – and of these, 268 people are indexed as medical practitioners. Entries are, of course, written individually, and the products are individual. But if we begin to look at them as a collective enterprise, what can we find?

It is possible to consider the making of national biographies such as the *ADB* from at least two complementary perspectives – either as a species of

Colonial doctors and national myths 129

writing, following certain conventions and editorial styles, intended to produce formulaic accounts in which the use of the adjectival and the anecdotal is limited – in which, therefore, authorial intent is difficult to discern – and in which limitations of space curtail narrative; and as a convenient means of packaging history, or qualifying history, following a consensual style that privileges the descriptive – that is, what can be generally agreed upon – over the problematic – that is, that which historians may debate. Entries in national biographies are to be informative, authoritative, definitive. Above all, they are to be factual. But on closer inspection, some of the images become as compelling as the facts. Between the lines of the *ADB*'s medical biographies emerge indications of what remains to be asked, rather than what should be assumed or taken as read, about Australian medical history.

These perspectives become clearer when we look at the three periods, written over two generations, in their description of three historical generations of Australian medical practitioners. One cannot divine editorial or authorial intent, but it is possible to detect certain underlying tonalities. In the first series – 1788–1850, in two volumes, written in 1966 and 1967 – the contributions made by colonial doctors to medical ideas and practice are rarely matters of principal focus. Their biographers included historians, not medical historians, familiar with colonial documents, and writing often from official accounts. Their language reflects the circumstances of hardship on the fringes of civilised settlement, and make summary judgements on the worthy and unworthy who found themselves in a place one biographer describes as 'sunk in crime, drunkenness and vice'.[12] The picture given of the first sixty-seven colonial doctors is compellingly bleak. From the 1780s to the 1820s, the transplanted practitioners found Australian life nasty and brutish, if not always short. From the First Fleet through the 1790s, medical men bound for Australia typically came as assistant naval surgeons.[13] Many enlisted for the Napoleonic Wars or the Indian service, and afterwards, to supplement their naval halfpay, found employment as surgeons – afterwards as surgeon-superintendents – on convict transports. Once in the colonies – either Norfolk Island, Van Diemen's Land or New South Wales – they were appointed to positions on land, sometimes moving several times before settling, or returning to England.

At the time, the usual way to qualify as a medical practitioner in the British Isles was to serve an apprenticeship, and then set up in practice, with or without passing an examination offered by the Society of Apothecaries, or the Royal Colleges of Surgeons of London or Edinburgh, or by taking a degree from a Scottish or continental University.[14] For the first seventy-five years of European settlement in Australia, formal qualifications were found only overseas.[15] What passed for colonial medical practice was a kind of general skill, which accepted but bypassed the tripartite class divisions of British medicine, much as did its American counterpart. For this reason, medical credentials are rarely a matter of comment.

Instead, we are introduced to the practitioners as people. Harsh life produced harsh manners, but also exposed the true nobility of 'natural gentlemen', whose badge was character, rather than birth. The *ADB* reminds us that not all early Australian medical men came by choice. Among those who did not, was William Redfern, Canadian-born, English-educated surgeon's mate – after whom the Sydney suburb is named – who was transported for his role in the ill-judged mutiny at Spithead, and who arrived in the colony without documents. Once his talents were discovered, he was examined and passed by three naval surgeons, who thus established a precedent for professional examinations in the colony – if only by a polite variation of a kangaroo court. Redfern then taught William Cooper, whom the *ADB* describes as Australia's first medical student, and in 1826 began what became a 'migratory momentum' in sending his son to Edinburgh to be medically educated.[16] In the meanwhile, Redfern acquired 23,000 acres, and if he 'lacked a gracious bedside manner', we are told, his 'experience and skill made ample amends for any apparent absence of overflowing politeness'.[17]

In a land briefly governed by Captain Bligh, it is not surprising that Redfern, the most notable of the early doctors, never forgot, nor was forgiven, his part in a naval mutiny. Nor were others absolved by their contemporaries, although they achieve *ADB* status – such as William Bland, founder of the *Australian Medical Journal*, and first president of the Australian Medical Association in 1859, who was transported for murder – and was denied a position on the newly-founded University Senate.[18] New South Wales did not end transportation until 1847, and even then proved reluctant to entrust its civic institutions – outside the police – to men, however well qualified, who had once worn convict arrows. Instead, it chose to celebrate them as men of low breeding, but good example. Thus the *ADB* includes John Irving, 'a convict bred to surgery', transported for larceny, who survived to demonstrate, in the *ADB*'s words, that 'universal depravity did not prevail'.[19] It was a point worthy of note in a history otherwise laden by opportunism and greed.

Fittingly, some few of the *ADB*'s medical men, whether convict or military, are remembered for their contributions to science, rather than medicine, recalling the close identification of naval surgeons and naturalists in narratives of British exploration. Colonial doctors were initially men of naval necessity, who – like Joseph Arnold, ship's surgeon on HMS *Victory*, and later naturalist to Raffles at Singapore – could identify with others whom the *ADB* counts as Australian, including Captain Cook. Later, their image reflects contemporary cockleshell heroes such as Flinders and Bass. Several accompany expeditions of inland or coastal exploration and collecting specimens that few Europeans had ever seen.[20] James Backhouse, naturalist and Quaker missionary of Tasmania, bequeathed volumes to Kew and his name to a genus. Arthur Smyth is remembered as the first white man to see an emu, and Joseph Milligan, Scottish-born secretary of the Royal Society of Van Dieman's Land, is included for his earliest studies of aboriginal languages, a work 'not free from error', we are told, 'but a remarkable achievement for a man who was said to be unacquainted with any language but English'.[21]

The first generations of colonial doctors were ubiquitous. Convict surgeons in the *ADB* treated officers and settlers, men and women, and even Aborigines on occasion, although some drew the line at midwifery. George Storey, educated in Edinburgh, arriving in 1829, found himself paid 3/s a day to be the district surgeon in Van Diemen's Land, to witness all floggings and postmortems, conduct vaccinations, inspect road gangs and make weather reports, as well as to treat families and assigned servants for illness, accidents and injuries from Aborigines. He also found time to become secretary of the Royal Society of Tasmania, superintendent of the Botanic Gardens, a specimen collector, and a leading Quaker.[22]

Badly paid, most received land grants in lieu of salary, and any temptation to focus on healing was overridden by the necessity to combine medicine with business. Whether convict or free settlers, many took convict wives and became pastoralists, founded banks, and set up joint stock companies. Frequently, entries read, 'surgeon naturalist and shipowner'; or 'surgeon and landholder' or – as for John Harris – 'surgeon, public servant and landowner'.[23] Few enough are cited for their institutional professional achievements: H. Grattan Douglas, one of the colony's first clinical teachers, led the movement in 1860 to require medical practitioners to have formal qualifications in medicine, surgery, and pharmacy.[24] But until the 1890s, most were content to let qualifications be decided in practice.

Qualifications for the first series, if rarely medical, are often political. The entry for Cornelius Casey – assistant colonial surgeon at Port Arthur in 1833, and grandfather of Lord Casey, the statesman – reminds us that 'men working together in isolated surroundings have difficulty in avoiding quarrels'. Homilectically we are reminded, many 'unpleasantnesses' resulted.[25] Some few – Cunningham was one – 'seems to have made no enemies even in Darling's NSW',[26] but the converse was more often true; and many seem to have won entries precisely because of their disputatious character. Thus we have James Hall, convicted of perjury, litigious and meddlesome, whose behaviour improved when he exchanged Botany Bay for Bermuda in 1826.[27]

In the 1830s, more doctors came to New South Wales as free settlers, many for reasons of their own health. One such was Thomas Cotter, 'callous and quarrelsome,' according to the ADB, and certainly the most controversial figure in the history of Adelaide's colonial infirmary.[28] Cotter's appointment as colonial surgeon in 1837 seems to have been the only evidence of planning for medical services in South Australia. He was told his duties would be 'exactly similar to those of a parish surgeon in England' – that is, his patients would come from the deserving poor, bearing chits from the resident commissioner – and like many a Poor Law Medical Officer in Dickensian England, his life was spent ordering food and protesting against bureaucratic niggardliness. Unlike his English counterparts, however, he diversified into property; and in the colonial idiom, lost his temper with the administration, was censured for neglect, both of his patients and the Port Augusta Literary Society he volunteered to run.[29] He was finally forced from office for having 'little patience with disappointed newcomers with imagined ailments or with malingering prisoners who demanded admission to the overcrowded surgery'.[30]

His near contemporary, John Coverdale, born in Bengal of a British postmaster, received his medical education in Glasgow, became a ship's doctor on the East India Company's transports, until he set upon a career in Tasmania. In 1836, he was given the combined job of colonial medical officer, warden of the gaol, keeper of the orphanage, and surgeon of Port Arthur's infamous penitentiary, where he looked after convicts, lunatics and imbeciles (last ship 1852) on a budget of £800 a year.[31] All confronted the colonial administration, and few in the main remained aloof from political intrigue.

Thus we meet Sir Robert Officer, 'medical officer and politician' – a nice tautology in the first half century of settlement – born in Dundee, and qualified by the Royal College of Surgeons of London, who suffered officially in 1831 for sending convict patients for treatment, saying he 'had no desire to be known as a mere slave driver', and thereby interfering with their discipline. He was an experimentalist with native oils and a reformer of city streets, exasperating even that most civic-minded of governors, Sir William Denison, to say that 'foul smell is indeed a nuisance but many people consider it a much greater nuisance to be made to pay for the remedy'. The *ADB* chose the Anglican *Church Times* to bestow the last blessing: 'he was a Presbyterian [they said] who knew nothing of Presbyterian prejudices'.[32] Charity of this sort began at home.

Few men of the first series became wealthy from medical practice, and no one could grow rich on a government salary.[33] D'Arcy Wentworth, Irish-born, who rates eight columns devoted to his family history in Armagh, ran away to the colonies to escape charges of robbery, and rapidly rose to become chief magistrate, controller of the Police Fund, and a founder of the Bank of New South Wales. 'Of no particular distinction as a medical officer', we are told, he was nonetheless conspicuous for fathering a large and influential family, and as keeping above the 'contentiousness and bickering' around him. Apologetically, the *ADB* commends him for his contribution to colonial life, 'whatever the irregularities of his private life'.[34] Alexander Collie, Edinburgh-trained doctor and world traveller, settled in Western Australia, and in 1834 built the best house in Perth, 'with bells hung and knocker up – rarities in this savage land'.[35] Sir Thomas Jamison, 'lived like a genteel and prosperous English squire, ultimately marrying the housekeeper by whom he had already had two sons and five daughters'.[36] A very few, like the generous Sir Charles Nicholson, were bound more by anglophile sentiments than Australian commitments, served their new country best by leaving it, and becoming one of the 'Australian colonial push in London'.[37]

In the first series, and reaching into the second – written by 1974 – value judgements seem to surface unexpectedly, like artesian springs in the outback. Patrick Cussen, 'a colourful character and an efficient public servant', is welcomed as a person 'well suited to be the first leader of his profession in a new settlement' (1839, first surgeon to operate in Victoria, first Public Vaccinator; and among first to use anaethesia).[38] On the other side, John Hampton, Edinburgh-trained surgeon and controller general of convicts, arrested on allegations of employing convicts for personal profit, is deemed worthy of inclusion, because his 'personal rule' intensified clamour for representative government and reform of convict management. Another victim turned success was James Bowman, inspector of colonial hospitals in 1828, who dabbled in 2,000 sheep and 12,000 acres, and became a director of the Bank of Australia, but who suffered heavy losses, in an experience that turned what Macarthur called a 'respectable prudent man' and competent surgeon into a victim of circumstance. 'Ambition, and the influence of MacArthur,' says his entry, 'led him from this field of sound achievement into activities which were beyond his ability to understand or control, and which, in the end, profited him nothing.'[39]

That nothing profited men, save unremitting sacrifice, appears a constant reminder of an Australia that recent immigrants find difficult to recognise, and image-merchants of Australia wish to forget. How many more were like Edward Luttrell, a private medical practitioner of Kent, who came to improve himself (and went?); who was rebuked by Macquarie (1813) for being 'criminally inattentive, totally undeserving, deficient in Humanity and in Attention to his Duty; sordid and unfeeling, [a man who] will not afford any medical assistance to any person who cannot pay him well for it'. Luttrell was kept on the colonial payroll – largely, it is said, for the sake of his large family.[40]

Some colonial doctors, almost forgotten by residents – Cunningham, Balmain, Redfern – left their names on rivers, stations, streets and suburbs. Others were not so lucky. At least ten were scoundrels and rogues, cashiered from their positions; others were sacked for reasons – such as a refusal to attend floggings – which admit of more than one interpretation. Some, few, are known for detesting brutality, but this is not an expectation, let alone reason for inclusion. One, Edward Barker, is described as combining gold digging with medicine – as if there were a natural affinity between the two.[41] A few prospered, but many did not, and six ended their lives in poverty or bankruptcy.

For most, a distinction between the public and private was at best arbitrary, at worst, inconvenient, and in any case, malleable. Facing overwhelming odds, their accomplishments, meagre, and their tools, before anaesthestics and antisepsis, very few. The best among them – including Thomas Reid, who detested brutalities – were judged 'humanitarian'.[42] Many turned their birthright and experience to civic improvements, and these the *ADB* singles out for special praise. Edward Hall, a 'young and fighting Irishman', not only 'loved to fight, but was praised for his untiring advocacy of health reforms aimed at assisting helpless children, and for the compulsory Vaccination Act that was being rushed through Parliament at his death'.[43] The role of medical men in the colonial march to representative government, was led, the *ADB* would have us believe, by such ordinary men, performing extraordinary deeds.

Whether men made the place, or the place made the men, the *ADB* leaves us to infer for ourselves; but the image given in the first series is a mixed picture of tribulation and turpitude, setback and survival – a canvass of human frailty and opportunity, qualified by embittered memories, and interrupted by occasional illuminations of science, humanity, and material success. Thus, Martin Mason – in 1804 the first medical practitioner to enter private practice – provoked a mutiny among convicts to protest against working conditions in the coal mines, and went on to suffer imprisonment for the sake of Governor Bligh at the hands of Macarthur during the Rum Rebellion – was redeemed by the *ADB*, as an ideal Australian type: 'blunt and dogmatic, harsh yet efficient [he] reflected, to a degree, the turbulent era of Australian history in which he lived'. Lacking subtlety, rejecting aristocratic pretences, he accepted the penal character of the colony for what it was, identified with appointed authority, and 'showed himself prepared to accept the consequences of his convictions'.[44]

Eurocentric, masculine, and almost without exception, ignorant of indigenous methods of treatment, to be colonial was to exist in two worlds – the world of the colonial appointment; and a world in which everything one did could be described as colonial. Nothing is assumed about his integrity or professional purpose. In the *ADB*, his image is mediated by a larger message – that of an environment, inner and outward, that is almost too hard to live with, that must be overcome, but that will never be overcome, at least not by Europeans; and what success men will have cannot be measured – although they are stated – in European terms. His language and customs are derivative of Britain, but are also reactions against it. His working life combines business, medical practice, politics, and commerce, frequently at the same time, and without apparent conflicts of interest. Public duty rarely interferes with private interest. This is the image of the colonial profession.

Is it also the image of colonial history? Perhaps, but as we look back at the *ADB*, we see different things. In the first series, written in the early 1960s, there are striking silences. Women, Aborigines, Europeans other than Britons do not feature prominently, nor among the medical entries. There is little sense of Europeans learning from the place or its native peoples. Instead, there is a sentiment that might be construed as favouring 'independence' of mind and action, mildly anti-British in its tradition, although qualified by acceptance of British models, adapted to local circumstance.

Thus, in 1808, the first examination of a man desiring to practice medicine, was, in the absence of any higher authority, conducted by three colonial surgeons acting as a jury of peers. Not until 1839 was a Medical Board established in New South Wales, and not until 1851 was there a medical school. Even then, there was disagreement about the value of a

European medical qualification unsupported by practical colonial experience. John Smith, the Dean of the Faculty of Medicine at Sydney University, actively opposes proposals to offer a medical degree in the colonial capital, on the grounds that qualified men are little different from quacks.[45] This is the new world, in which all is cast in doubt.

It is also, however, biography, and interpretations are left to history. As we move from the first series to the second and third – that is, to 1850–1890 and 1890–1939 – we encounter subtle shifts – and articles wider in editorial range, choice of subjects, and choice of treatment. Authors also change, as increasingly an earlier tradition of amateurs and local historians is overtaken, or complemented, by a new generation of academic historians and medical practitioners, some of whom – especially in more recent volumes – seem to have personal knowledge of their subjects. Colonial physicians and surgeons were neither cut in marble, nor, as Mr Fairbrother assured Mr Causabon, were they stone effigies. But by the late 1970s, more space is given to their credentials, and less to their foibles.

By the late 1970s and early 1980s, more academic historians, trained in social history, appear to have joined the authorial team, bringing new questions to their material. Overall, it seems that the imperatives of national history, reaching beyond colonial nationalism, are pressing. Mixing with Kipling – conservative and anglophile imperialists, are radicals and republicans, the 'national type' – the Coming Men of the 1890s and the 1990s, the archetypes of popular literature, mass literacy and democracy – a medical presence in the march to nationhood.[46] Thus, George Adam, born in Leeds, who migrates to Victoria and introduces antisepsis into obstetrics, is cited for his contribution to Australian golf.[47] Robert Allan, 'no seeker after hollow status', is commended for his service to King and Empire in the Australian Imperial Forces (AIF) at Gallipoli, in Mesopotamia, and in France – and is parenthetically thanked for introducing a diploma of obstetrics and gynaecology to Australia in 1932.[48]

In the second series, four volumes between 1969 and 1976, there are only eighty-one medical entries. Familiar verities – the perils of doubtful success in an uncertain world – continue to feature prominently. Doctors are among the victims of Australian conditions. Henry Armit, editor of the *Medical Journal of Australia*, despite an 'imposing presence and costly manner', 'died in poverty and left his family in debt'[49] – a setback written in language many Australians of a certain age will recognise. Yet, the list is quixotic, if not eccentric. How are we to account for the appearance, indexed as a medical practitioner, of Mahomet Allum – camel driver, herbalist, and philanthropist of Adelaide – who flourished in the 1920s – a period when, we are told, 'dissatisfaction with conventional medical practice was enabling herbalists and faith healers to flourish'.[50]

Alas, Allum is not typical. And as we move into the third series – six volumes, and 220 medical entries, written between 1979–1990 – the emphasis changes. In some ways, it becomes more predictable. What constitutes an 'admissible' candidate and an acceptable entry seems to adapt to new circumstances. By the third series, all entries are Australian born, a though many continue to receive part or all of their education overseas. Men of action are for the first time joined by women of action – some twenty-nine before the series ends. There is less attention given to 'extra-curricular' activities, and more to medical careers.

In part, this may well reflect the tenor of Australian history, as the bricolage of colonial employment settles into more orderly professional life. Indeed, whilst entries still speak of business interests outside medicine, these are narrated as career moves, rather than as commitments. On the face of it, the medical profession of the 1930s, 1940s, and 1950s possessed fewer scoundrels, rogues, and bankrupts than ever before; and by the late 1950s, all such had entirely disappeared. Few, if any, modern medical men spent any time as guests of His Majesty, ended their lives in poverty, or left their families in distress. Few, if any, were born illegitimate, and none had private lives to speak of, except those typically summarised in the inevitability polite, closing mention of surviving wives and children.

By the close of the third series, in the late 1980s, accounts of worthy achievements almost completely replace colonial misdemeanors and business intrigues. War service weighs significantly – of the 220 medical practitioners, 66 have military experience in one or both world wars. Personal assessments, where they appear, are no less judgemental, but they appear more qualified. Richard Arthur, social reformer and practitioner, who campaigned against Britain in the South African war, and fought for federal child endowment in the 1920s, Michael Roe describes as 'held in real, if somewhat patronising, affection'.[51] Tall poppies, like Robert Stopford, stand as beacons of worthiness, but whether he is in any way typical of his era, we are left unsure.[52] Individuals are just individuals, and their roles as historical actors, or national types, are less well developed. On the contrary, authorial comment highlights uniqueness, rather than typicality. Or so one would hope. Consider Clive Shields, Victorian-born medical practitioner and practical man, sometime Minister of Agriculture and Mines, who became disillusioned with voters who apparently cared nothing for democracy. What the country needed, he said in 1938, was 'a taste of dictatorship'.[53]

Biography illuminates the collective, by focusing light on the individual. But whether we are safe to read patterns of history through these lives remains unclear. What in the first series appear as heroic, if flawed, stereotypes, towards the end appear as worthy citizens. Perhaps we are on safer ground if we view entries more as snapshots, bearing in mind that the camera never lies.

Medical biography and colonial stereotypes

Elsewhere, I have discussed five stereotypes that have come to characterise colonial science in Australia.[54] These, I have suggested, are (1) the persistence of an amateur naturalist tradition; (2) an enduring culture of critical scepticism; (3) an enveloping 'cult of practicality'; (4) a deep-seated recognition of the fragility of European life, subject always to a harsh and threatening natural environment; and (5) the acceptance of an economy governed by 'boom and bust', which harbours a more than even prospect of loss than gain. In the first century of settlement, these categories can be extended to colonial doctors; to whom we can add three more: a close engagement with political and government life, active intervention in property and commerce, and a close participation in civic development. For those of appropriate age and service, the *ADB* recognised military achievement, as well as medical prowess. There could be a reasonable expectation that Australian doctors would mend limbs, deliver babies, heal the sick, and bring the blessings of humanity to the community – but such issues rarely figure in the first two series, and are only hinted at in the third.

Alongside the doctors, the *ADB* tells us of Morton Allport, naturalist and solicitor of Hobart, an authority on acclimatisation who collected the Fellowship of the Linnean, and of the zoological societies of London and Brussels. William Archer – 'architect, naturalist, landowner and politician' used science much as a rising man might in Dalton's Manchester, or Hooker's Kew, in collecting and sending plants home, becoming known as 'a useful man for Tasmania' – although, as the *ADB* sadly relates, 'he could have been much more'.

The implication that to be more, to do more, would be rewarded with posthumous fame, is an underlying subtext. Industry was to be as important for the colonial doctor as intellect. And nothing in life so honoured a man as his passing – in the Australian epic, preferably from exhaustion and dysentery. This message of honorable death is written in many colonial lives. The *ADB* would be incomplete without Edmund Kennedy (1818–1848), plagued by insects and Aborigines, or the high-souled Wills, dying before the aptly named Mt Hopeless, or the tragic John Gilbert, ornithologist, whose marmoreal monument in Edmund Blackett's neo-Georgian St James's Church in Sydney takes as its motto the Horacian paraphrase, *Dulci et decorum est pro Scientia mori* (A classically virtuous death unites men of science and medicine). But, as Peter Carey puts it, death is a quintessentially local act. Australian history, seen through the first series, begins with doctors enduring a culture of defeat. With this comes an image of downgraded success, in which defeat is the expectation, and failure all too often the norm. In this looking glass world, Alice's race of the Dodos is stood on its head: medical practice becomes a race in which nobody wins.

Through the second series – covering 1850–1890, and written between 1969–1976 – this sentiment associates colonial doctors with the 'cult of practicality'. Medical men reflect the national type – the 'practical man' – born in England, but brought to bloom in Australia. The typical doctor appears in the pages of Marcus Clarke in 1877:

> A square-headed, masterful man, with full temples, plenty of beard, a keen eye, a stern and yet sensual mouth. His teeth will be bad and his lungs good. He will suffer from liver disease, and become prematurely bald. . . . His religion will be a form of Presbyterianism; his national policy a democracy tempered by the rate of exchange.[55]

Substitute Presbyterian Scots for Irish, and we have an almost universal image of ingenuity, self-reliance, and masculine Australian-ness. As Charles Bean, Gallipoli war correspondent and founder of the Australian War Memorial, wrote his editor at the *Sydney Morning Herald*:

> It is still a quality of the Australian that he can make something out of nothing . . . he has to do without the best things, because they don't exist there. So he has made the next best do; and, where even these are not to hand, he has manufactured them out of things which one would have thought impossible to turn to any use at all. He has done it for so long that it has become more than an art. It has long since become part of his character, the most valuable part of it.[56]

For the practical man of medicine, the tyrannies of isolation were facts of life that counted for more than credentials. Living in Australia was, for about a third of the medical entries, not enough, and early colonial lives show a tendency to return to Britain physically, or never leave it spiritually. Those who remain in Australia become part of the establishment. 'Theirs was the world of the male, protestant, imperial clerisy',[57] and their successors joined the conservative class. Eventually, the limitations of colonial medical practice were overcome – if not until the late 1940s – or so we may infer from entries written in the late 1980s. As we move into volume 14, in the series newly begun, we will see whether such hopeful anticipations were realised, and what profiles will be given those who flourished since 1940 and gave Australian medicine its post-colonial present.

Conclusion

Looking at Australia's standard reference work dedicated to national biography inevitably prompts questions about the writing of Australian medical lives. How does the *ADB* portray colonial medicine and the later medical biography of Australia? Does it offer a reliable purchase on the leading characteristics of Australian medicine? Whose history is being written? To such questions, I can offer no definitive answers. But I would suggest that, in using the *ADB*, certain caveats should apply. In supplying certain kinds of facts, it can be relied upon. And in restoring the Australian past from what W. E. H. Stanner called the 'national cult of forgetting',[58] the *ADB* has played a magnificent role. But as a source of interpretations, it cannot do other than reflect the conditions of authorship and direction under which it was written. Perhaps inevitably, the *ADB* has helped establish stereotypes of 'Australianness' that may not escape unchallenged by the coming generation.

In the coming decades, we are certain to see Australian biography moving away from images dominated by a European past and by negotiations with that past; and reaching towards men and women of different backgrounds, operating within local environments, representing a wider range of ethnic origins, and conveying a more equitable gender balance. We are beginning to find room for Georgiana Molloy, Louisa Atkinson, Louisa Meredith, Elizabeth Gould, Lady Jane Franklin, and Fanny Macleay, and explorers such as Ellis Rowan and Amalie Dietrich. William Lines suggests that colonial women defined themselves not by their involvement in 'science', but rather in the gendered space assigned to natural history, where they could privilege particular ways of knowing.[59] Until it remedies this, the *ADB* must fail to be a dictionary of truly 'national' biography.

Historians of science have not been slow to see the point. In Canberra, Tim Sherrat, working from the Australian Scientific Archives Project (ASAP) embassy at the Australian Academy of Science, has introduced 'Bright SPARCS' – a World Wide Web resource, which includes information on about 2,000 Australian scientific men and women from the eighteenth century to the present. This database grew from RASA (Register of the Archives of Science in Australia), and is still growing, a tribute to Rod Home's bibliography of Australian physics and subsequent additions. So far, this project is drawing together existing material, and making it more widely available in electronic form. But a larger subtext is emerging, as it creates a new biographical dictionary of Australian science, forming a reservoir of data for Australian historians, school teachers, and pupils.

If, as I have argued, we are approaching a cusp in the curve, or the curl of a wave, in the history of colonial biography, it is possible to suggest some lines along which work might now proceed. At one level, the reading public is still interested in 'fairy tales of science'. In this, the sheer account of much negotiation with nature that lies hidden within the *ADB*, and much that is not, will easily furnish a bay of books. But as professional historians of science, who turn to biography as a narrative form, as well as to literary historians and writers who see in science a rich cultural resource, it is useful to unpackage and reconstruct the past, not to produce improving literature, but critical accounts of the pursuit of natural knowledge in colonial conditions – an enterprise, flawed, often compromised, sometimes destined to failure.

On theoretical grounds, we have a choice: on an optimistic reading, science biographers can co-opt the new historicism, reducing false boundaries between disciplines, and reading lives as texts. Or else we can simply wait until the postmodernist wave passes, like a tropical storm in the Coral Sea, or a southerly buster rushing up from the Antarctic, leaving behind it the remains of a long narrative tradition. Manning Clark was deeply concerned –

obsessed – with binaries – the bane of postmodern theorists – and his history reverberates to the drums of measurers and levellers, men and women, lovers and believers, bush and city, civilisation and barbarism. So, too, we have the legacy of Patrick White's preoccupation with the individual confronted with Bunsen's trilogy of god, man, and humanity. It was difficult in the past to see how scientific biography can fit comfortably into a tradition of binaries, as its role is precisely that of mediator – between ideas and actions, internalist and externalist, abstract and concrete, objectivity and subjectivity, concept and application. For this reason, we require modern tools of interpretive flexibility, to look again at the traffic in ideas between the traditional binaries of metropolis and periphery, the self and the other.

This, however, is to read ahead. Just as to read *Ulyssees* is to see how an Irishman took the language of the invader and turned it against him, so to read Australian biography today is to see how an agenda is slowly shifting away from a colonial past, and towards new, contested meanings, among a population that is increasingly multicultural, and not yet sure of the identity it should, or does, have at the beginning of the millennium and the centenary of Federation. The burden of stereotypes can be suffocating; secondary sources are inevitably prejudiced by the official past; and much will have to be unwritten, before it is written again. Biography gives us an opportunity to re-value, and if necessary, reconfirm, the myths of the bush, the legend of the outback, instead of letting repeated mention of cult phrases become a substitute for examining them. At the beginning of the millennium, possibly sooner than its founders imagined, the *ADB* may have to reflect upon its own history, and revisit the images it has created. Whether those images are typical – or if not, whose interests precisely they represent – are questions historians need to know. In giving space to medical biography, *ADB* offers a window upon Australian medical history, helping us to find and engage with Australian lives, and not merely tell them. But to re-examine the ways in which it has told those lives is, in my view, a need whose time has come.

Acknowledgement

*   An earlier version of this chapter was presented to the conference on 'Medicine and the Colonies', convened by the Society for the Social History of Medicine, and held at Oxford in July 1996. The present formulation owes much to generous comments received at that time. I am also grateful to Dr Laurence Geary of University College, Cork, for access to his continuing work on Scottish and Irish doctors in Australia; and to Dr Chris Cuneen, of the *Australian Dictionary of Biography*, for his ever helpful suggestions.

Notes

1 Michael Holroyd, quoting Philip Guedalla, in 'Literary and Historical Biography,' in Anthony M. Friedson (ed.), *New Directions in Biography*, Honolulu, University of Hawaii Press, pp. 12–25 at 23. The quotation is drawn from an

Colonial doctors and national myths 141

address on literary biography given by Guedalla in 1929. A different version of the quotation was used by Sir Oliver Lodge in 'The New Outlook in Physics', *Discovery*, 1929, vol. X, no. 109.
2 Quoted in Gerald Searle, *From Deserts the Prophets Come: The Creative Spirit in Australia, 1788–1972*, Melbourne, Heinemann, 1973, p. 56.
3 I am indebted for this information to Mr Laurie Carlson of Deakin University, who has since 1981 heroically produced annual bibliographical supplements for the *Historical Records of Australian Science*.
4 Cf. David Knight, *Humphry Davy: Science and Power*, London, Blackwell, 1992.
5 Martin Ince, 'Genius for Sale: From 2p per Savant', *Times Higher*, 19 August 1994, p. 21, reviewing Trevor Williams (ed.), *Collins Biographical Dictionary of Scientists*, London, HarperCollins, 1994; Roy Porter (ed.), *The Hutchinson Dictionary of Scientific Biography*, London, Hutchinson, 1994; and Hazel Muir (ed.), *Larousse Dictionary of Scientists*, Paris, Larousse, 1994.
6 Joy Hooton, 'Australian Autobiography and the Question of National Identity: Patrick White, Barry Humphries, and Manning Clark', *A/B: Auto/Biography Studies*, 1994, vol. 9, no. 1, pp. 43–63, at 51.
7 Patrick White, quoted in Peter Ward, 'White the Warrior', *The Weekend Australian*, 30 April–1 May 1988, p. 9.
8 Quoted in James Walter, 'Biography, Psychobiography and Cultural Space', in Ian Donaldson (ed.), *Shaping Lives: Reflections on Biography*, Canberra, ANU, 1992, p. 260.
9 Walter, op. cit., p. 286.
10 Manning Clark, *Making History*, vol. 66, cited in Hooton, op. cit., p. 61.
11 Preface to *Australian Dictionary of Biography*, vol. 13 (1940–1980), pp. v–vi.
12 B. H. Fletcher, 'Thomas Arndell (1753–1821)', *ADB*, 1966, vol. i, pp. 27–8.
13 J. Hooke, 'The Adelaide Hospital from Foundation to Federation: A Case Study in the Factors Shaping Medical Publication in a Transplanted Society, 1836–1900 – A Bibliography in Context', Adelaide, np, 1991, vol. 1, p. 52, cited in Bernard Nicholson, 'Thomas Young Cotter – Colonial Surgeon, South Australia, Success or Failure?', in Susanne Atkins *et al.*, *Outpost Medicine*, Hobart, University of Tasmania, 1994, pp. 283–94.
14 P. Rhodes, *An Outline History of Medicine*, London, Butterworth, 1985, p. 114.
15 Laurence M. Geary, 'The Scottish–Australian Connection, 1850–1900', in Vivian Nutton and Roy Porter (eds), *The History of Medical Education in Britain*, Amsterdam, Rodopi, 1995, p. 52.
16 Geary, op. cit., p. 57.
17 Edward Ford, 'William Redfern (1774?–1868)', *ADB*, 1967, vol. ii, pp. 368–71.
18 John Cobley, 'William Bland (1789–1868)', *ADB*, 1966, vol. i, pp. 112–15.
19 A. J. Gray, 'John Irving (d. 1795)', *ADB*, 1967, vol. ii, pp. 4–5.
20 Charles Bateson, 'Joseph Arnold (1782–1818)', *ADB*, 1966, vol. i, p. 29; Keith Macrae Bowden, 'George Bass (1771–1803)', *ADB*, 1966, vol. i, pp. 64–5; John Cobley, 'William Bland (1789–1868)', *ADB*, 1966, vol. i, pp. 112–15.
21 Anon, 'Arthur Bowles Smyth (1750–1790)', *ADB*, 1967, vol. ii, pp. 453–4; W. G. Hoddinott, 'Joseph Milligan (1807–1884)', *ADB*, 1967, vol. ii, pp. 230–1.
22 Mary Bartram Trott, 'George F. Storey (1800–1885)', *ADB*, 1967, vol. ii, pp. 490–1.
23 George F. J. Bergman, 'John Harris (1783–1865)', *ADB*, 1966, vol. i, pp. 517–18.
24 K. B. Noad, 'Henry Douglass (1790–1865)', *ADB*, 1966, vol. i, pp. 314–16.
25 F. C. Green, 'Cornelius G. Casey (1810–1896)', *ADB*, 1966, vol. i, pp. 213–14.
26 L. F. Fitzhardinge, 'Peter Miller Cunningham (1789–1864)', *ADB*, 1966, vol. i, pp. 267–8.

27 Charles Bateson, 'James Hall (b. 1784)', *ADB*, 1966, vol. i, p. 503.
28 J. E. Hughes, *A History of the Royal Adelaide Hospital*, Adelaide, 1967, p. 6.
29 A. A. Lendon, 'Thomas Young Cotter, LCA, The First Colonial Surgeon for South Australia', Adelaide, Mortlock Library, n. d., p. 1.
30 Anon., 'Thomas Young Cotter (1805–1882)', *ADB*, 1966, vol. i, p. 248.
31 G. F. Sorell, 'John Coverdale (1814–1896)', *ADB*, 1966, vol. i, pp. 253–4; see also Susanne Atkins, 'Dr John Coverdale, 1814–1896, The Last Civil Commandant and Medical Officer of the Convict Settlement of Port Arthur, 1873–1877', in Susanne Atkins et al., *Outpost Medicine*, pp. 295–301.
32 Anon., 'Sir Robert Officer (1800–1879)', *ADB*, 1967, vol. ii, pp. 297–8.
33 G. H. Stancombe, 'James Scott (1790–1837)', *ADB*, 1967, vol. ii, pp. 427–8.
34 J. J. Auchmuty, 'D'Arcy Wentworth (1762?–1827)', *ADB*, 1967, vol. ii, pp. 579–82.
35 B. C. Cohen, 'Alexander Collie (1793–1844)', *ADB*, 1966, vol. i, pp. 235–6.
36 Vivienne Parsons, 'Thomas Jamison (1745–1811)', *ADB*, 1967, vol. ii, pp. 12–13.
37 David S. Macmillan, 'Sir Charles Nicholson (1808–1903)', *ADB*, 1967, vol. ii, pp. 283–5.
38 Bryan Gandevia, 'Patrick Cussen (1792–1849)', *ADB*, 1966, vol. i, pp. 272–3.
39 B. H. Fletcher, 'James Bowman (1763–1825)', *ADB*, 1966, vol. i, pp. 138–9.
40 Anon., 'Edward Luttrell (1756–1824)', *ADB*, 1967, vol. ii, pp. 139–40.
41 K. F. Russel, 'Edward Barker 1816–1885', *ADB*, 1969, vol. iii, pp. 89–90.
42 Charles Bateson, 'Thomas Reid (1791–1825)', *ADB*, 1967, vol. ii, p. 376.
43 Anon., 'Edward Hall (1805–1881)', *ADB*, 1966, vol. i, pp. 502–3.
44 T. W. Blunden, 'Martin Mason (d. 1821)', *ADB*, 1967, vol. ii, pp. 213–14.
45 Milton Lewis, 'The Medical Profession and Professor Smith', in Roy MacLeod (ed.), *University and Community in Nineteenth Century Sydney: Professor John Smith (1821–1885)*, Sydney, Sydney University Press, 1988, pp. 60–9.
46 Richard White, *Inventing Australia: Images and Identity, 1688–1980* (Sydney: George Allen and Unwin, 1981).
47 Frank M. C. Forster, 'George Rothwell Wilson Adam (1853–1924)', *ADB*, 1979, vol. vii, pp. 8–9.
48 Frank M. C. Forster, 'Robert Marshall Allan (1886–1946)', *ADB*, 1979, vol. vii, pp. 37–9.
49 W. L. Calov, 'Henry Armit (1870–1930)', *ADB*, 1979, vol. vii, p. 95.
50 Valmai A. Hankel, 'Mahomet Allum (1858?–1964)', *ADB*, 1979, vol. vii, p. 47.
51 Michael Roe, 'Richard Arthur (1865–1932)', *ADB*, 1979, vol. vii, pp. 103–4.
52 Stephen Garton, 'Robert Stopford (1862–1926)', *ADB*, 1990, vol. xii, p. 105.
53 Geoff Browne, 'Clive Shields (1879–1965)', *ADB*, 1988, vol. xi, pp. 593–4.
54 Roy MacLeod, 'The "Practical Man": Myth and Metaphor in Anglo-Australian Science', *Australian Cultural History*, no. 8, 1989, pp. 24–49.
55 Marcus Clarke, cited in Turner, *The Australian Dream*, cited in White, op. cit., p. 63.
56 Cited in M. Geissler, 'McAlpine Collection Goes on Display', *Australian Collector's Quarterly*, February–April, 1990, p. 12, and quoted in Kylie Winkworth, 'The Market and the Museum', in John Rickard and Peter Spearritt (eds), *Packaging the Past*, Melbourne, Melbourne University Press, 1991, p. 120.
57 F. B. Smith, 'Academics In and Out of the *Australian Dictionary of Biography*', in F. B. Smith and P. Crichton (eds), *Ideas for Histories of Universities in Australia* (Canberra: Australian National University, 1990), 9.
58 Hooton, op. cit., p. 60.
59 William Lines, *An All-Consuming Passion: Origins, Modernity, and the Australian Life of Georgiana Molloy* (St Leonards, NSW: Allen & Unwin, 1994). I am indebted for this point to Ms Claire Hooker.

Index

Aborigines: Aborigines Act (1905) 117; compulsory medical treatment 110, 117, 118, 119, 120; dependency, colonial construction of 112, 113; education 114; healthcare policies 112, 113, 114, 116–18; healthcare, resistance to 120; identity, self-determination of 109, 110; influenza epidemics 113, 118, 119; introduced diseases, effects of 107, 113, 114, 118, 119; leprosy 113, 115, 117, 118; malaria, effects of 113; medicine's role in the construction of colonial identities 9–10, 104, 109, 111–12, 114, 115, 120; mortality rates 113, 114; segregationist colonial policies 110, 115, 118, 119, 120; settler health, perceived threat to 9–10, 114, 115, 116; the stolen generation 103; tuberculosis epidemics 113; venereal diseases, spread of 110, 113, 116–17; see also Australia

amagqirha 41, 44, 48, 53; see also Xhosa

Arya Samaj: vernacular language schools 31–2

Australia: Aborigines Act (1905) 117; Advisory Council on Nutrition 89; Australian Scientific Archives Project 139; Australian Society for the History of Medicine 126; biography, historiography of 125, 126, 127, 138–40; colonial education policy 114; colonial health policies 105, 112, 113, 114, 116–18; colonial identities, medicine's role in the construction of 9–10, 104, 109, 111–12, 114, 115, 120, 121; colonial medicine, qualifying credentials 129, 131, 134–5; colonial medicine, service conditions 129, 131, 132; colonial science, stereotypes of 136–7; Institute of Tropical Medicine 9, 106, 107, 112; Medical Boards, establishment of 134; Rum Rebellion 134; segregationist colonial policies 110, 115, 118, 119, 120; tropical medicine and colonial identity 9–10, 106, 119, 121; tropical medicine, its implication in colonialism 106, 114, 115, 116; see also Aborigines, Australian Dictionary of Biography, Northern Territory, Queensland

Australian Dictionary of Biography: Aborigines, absence of 134, 139; colonial history, portrayal of 134; colonial medical biographies 10, 129–38; colonial medicine, portrayal of 129, 134, 135, 136, 137, 138; entry qualifications 130, 131, 135–6; honourable deaths 137; identity, construction of 138–9; military achievement, recognition of 135, 136, 137; origins of 128; purpose 128; scientific achievement, recognition of 130–1, 137; women, absence of 134, 139

Australian Society for the History of Medicine 126

Index

Ayurvedic medicine 6–7; All-India Ayurvedic Congress 26; dissemination of 22–4; origins of 14; revitalisation of 26–7, 33; see also *Stri Darpan*

Baine, B.: King William's Town Hospital, modernisation of 54
Bean, Charles 138
Bell, Muriel 91, 94
Breinl, A. 107, 112, 114
British Kaffraria 45, 46; annexation of 53; see also King William's Town Hospital

Cattle-Killing movement 46, 47, 51, 52
Christchurch: Britishness of 93; milk policy 92–4
Cilento, R. 112, 115, 118
Clifford, J. 3, 4
colonialism: colonial identities, medicine's role in the construction of 6–7, 9–10, 15, 104, 109, 111–12, 114, 115, 120, 121; hegemony, medicine's implication in 41, 42, 45–6, 61, 74, 106, 114, 115, 116; Indian nationalist identity, medicine's role in the construction of 6–7, 15, 22, 24, 33–4
Cook, Cecil 115, 118
cults of affliction 43, 44, 48; see also Xhosa

Dar, S. M. L. 29
Das, S. 27
Denison, William 132
Dulari, Prem 23, 27
Dutch East Indies: European midwives 71–3; indigenous midwifery 66, 67, 68, 69–70, 72; maternal mortality 70–1; midwifery reform 8, 62, 65–8, 71, 73; midwifery schools, establishment of 66; Society for the Improvement of Native Nursing 68

Elkington, J. S. C. 106, 112, 116

Fitzgerald, J. P. 7, 41; African doctors, training of 53–4; civilising mission 45–6, 49, 53; famine relief 51–2; Gota, relationship with 49; King William's Town Hospital, management of 49–50; nutrition, importance to 50; ophthalmia, treatment of 43, 47; vaccination program 50; Xhosa, attitude towards 46–7; Xhosa medicine, influence on 48, 53; Xhosa medicine, record of 43; see also Xhosa

Foucault, M. 1, 2, 4, 80

Gandhi, Mahatma 17, 18; Hindi Literature Conference, chairing of 21
Garg, M. 29
Glaxo 86–7
Gota 41, 48; Fitzgerald, relationship with 49; western medicine, use of 48; see also Xhosa
Gramsci, A. 2
Grey, G. 41, 42; African medicine, suppression of 44, 45, 53; British Kaffraria, governorship of 45; civilising mission 53; famine relief, prevention of 51; New Zealand, governorship of 45
Guha, R. 2, 3
Gurtu, J. 30

Hall, S. 6
Hasluck, P. 111, 114, 119
Heerlen school 64, 65, 71, 73
Horton, R. 47–8
Huggins, J. 109

identity: Cartesian self 1; colonial identities, medicine's role in the construction of 6–7, 9–10, 15, 104, 109, 111–12, 114, 115, 120, 121; gender 1; group 1; Indian nationalist identity, medicine's role in the construction of 6–7, 15, 22, 24, 33–4; individual 1; negotiation of 2, 4–5; reification of 4–5; self-determination of 2, 109, 110
igqirha 41, 43, 44, 47, 48, 53; see also Xhosa

India: Arya Samaj language schools 31–2; Ayurvedic medicine 6–7, 14, 22–4, 26–7, 33; child marriage, nationalist critique of 31; colonial dictionaries 20; Hindi prose, development of 20–2; infant mortality 30; maternal mortality 30; Matsya Purana 29; Medical Registration Acts 26–7; medicine and the construction of British colonial identity 15; medicine, codification of 30; midwifery expertise, loss of 30; nationalist identity, medicine's role in the construction of 6–7, 15, 22, 24, 33–4; Prayag Mahili Samiti 17, 19; *Sarasvati* 21; subaltern histories 2–3; traditional medicine, colonial suppression of 22; Unani medical texts 14; Western medicine, dissemination of 14–15, 22, 24–5; women's healthcare roles 27, 28, 30, 31, 32; the women's question 19, 20; *see also Stri Darpan*

Institute of Tropical Medicine 9, 106, 107, 112

Java *see* Dutch East Indies
Jha, P. 30
Jordan, D. 110

King William's Town Hospital 41, 45; funding of 53; hygiene regime 49–50; management of 49–50; modernisation of 54; mortality rates 50, 51; racial segregation 54; *see also* Fitzgerald
King, Truby 85, 87, 87
Kinsella, J. A. 92

Lawson, H.: advice to Australian writers 125
Leavitt, J. 5, 10
Levi-Strauss, C. 80

Macleod, R. 104, 105, 108
Maqoma, N. 49
Marcus, G. 3, 4

Matsya Purana: hygiene and health recommendations 29
medicine: civilising mission 45–6, 116; and colonial hegemony 41, 42, 45–6, 61, 74, 106, 106, 114, 115, 116; colonial identities, its role in the construction of 6–7, 9–10, 15, 104, 109, 111–12, 114, 115, 120, 121; Indian nationalist identity, its role in the construction of 6–7, 15, 22, 24, 33–4; pluralism 6; *see also* tropical medicine
Meuleman, Clemens 64, 65
midwifery: Dutch East Indies 8, 66, 67, 68, 69–73; Heerlen school 64, 65, 71, 72, 73; India 30; Netherlands 8, 62, 63, 64–5, 68, 71, 72; reform of 8, 62, 65–8, 71, 73; Society for the Improvement of Native Nursing 68
milk: and children's physical development 87–9; cultural symbolism 8–9, 80, 81, 84, 86, 95; dried milk and baby feeding debate 87; as medicine 88–9; school milk, state provision of 89–90, 91, 94; *see also* New Zealand
The Mirror of Women *see Stri Darpan*
Mitra, B. K. 23, 30
Mothercraft Training Centre 86
Mukandilal, Shriyut 24–5

Nehru, Jawaharlal 17
Nehru, Rameshwari 6, 15; Age of Consent Committee, work on 17; Ayurvedic medicine, promotion of 23, 24; editorial policy 18, 19; education of 17; family history 16, 17; nationalist women's organisations, involvement with 17; *see also Stri Darpan*
Nehru, Uma 18
Netherlands: Catholic childcare practices 64, 66; Catholicism, effects on midwifery 63, 64, 65, 72; Health Acts 63; Heerlen school 64, 65, 71, 72, 73; infant mortality 63; maternal mortality 71; midwifery and superstition 68; midwifery reforms 8, 62, 63, 64–5, 68, 71; southern

provinces, poverty of 62, 63, 73; southern provinces, social problems of 64

New Zealand: 'building Britons' 81; Central Milk Council 81, 93; Christchurch, milk policy 92–4; dairy produce, promotion of 82–3; dried milk exports 87; economic dependence on the United Kingdom 79, 80, 82, 83; Empire's Dairy Farm 82; Fernleaf 82; Glaxo, rise of 86–7; infant welfare 85–6; Karitane hospitals 86; Karitane Products 87; Maori children's diet 89; Milk Act 90; milk, adult consumption of 95; milk, apathy to 92; milk, 'building bodies' 95; milk, cultural symbolism 8–9, 80, 81, 84, 86, 95; milk, and infant welfare 85, 86, 87, 88, 89; milk, inspection of 90, 91, 92; milk, as medicine 88–9; Plunket Society 85, 87, 90; Primary Products Marketing Act (1936) 89; school milk, state provision of 89–90, 91, 94; settler identity, construction of 79, 80; United Kingdom's entry into the EEC, effect of on dairy industry 96; wartime commandeering of dairy produce 82–3, 90–1; Women's Food Value League 91

Nongqawuse: Cattle-Killing movement 46, 47, 51, 52

Northern Territory: Aborigines, quarantining of 110, 119; colonial identity, construction of 109, 111–12; leprosy 118; segregationist colonial policy 110, 119; tropical medicine, racist imperatives of 108; Venereal Disease Ordinances 110, 117–18; *see also* Aborigines, Australia

Plunket Society 85, 87, 90
Prayag Mahili Samiti 17, 19

Queensland: Leprosy Act (1892) 117; venereal diseases, spread of 116–17; *see also* Australia

Rickard, J. 127

Sarasvati: and the development of Hindi prose 21
Shukla, S. J. 24
South Africa 7; Ninth Frontier War 53; *see also* British Kaffraria, Xhosa
Stri Darpan: anatomy, promotion of 25–6; Ayurvedic medicine, dissemination of 22–4; childcare methods, promotion of 24–5; dual model of medicine, promotion of 22, 26, 27, 30, 31, 33; editorial policy 18, 19; exercise, promotion of 31; germ theory, dissemination of 26; healthcare, promotion of 6–7, 18; hygiene and disapproval of female Westernisation 28–30; medical ignorance, assumption of 27, 28, 30; medicine and the construction of nationalist identity 6–7, 15, 22, 24, 33–4; nationalist women's consciousness, communication of 18, 19; pedagogical mission of 18, 22, 27–8; purdah, critique of 30, 31; readership, class background of 6, 15–16, 21; tuberculosis, recommended treatment 29; Western medicine, dissemination of 14–15, 22, 24–5; women's identity, construction of 31; women's healthcare roles 27, 28, 30, 31, 32; women's movements, importance to 18, 19
subaltern histories 2–3

Tandon, K. N. 31
Tripathi Shrikant 24, 25
tropical medicine: civilising mission 116; colonial identity, its role in the construction of 9–10, 104, 119, 121; colonialism, its implication in 105, 106, 114, 115, 116; historiography 104–5; Institute of Tropical Medicine 9, 106, 107, 112; racist imperatives of 108

United Kingdom: dried milk imports 87; EEC entry 80, 96; imperial preference, opposition to 83; infant welfare 84, 85; Mothercraft Training Centre 86; New Zealand dairy produce, reliance on 82–3; New Zealand milk, inspection of 90; New Zealand's economic dependence on 79, 80, 82, 83; wartime commandeering of dairy produce 82–3, 90–1

Women's Food Value League 91
Worboys, M. 105, 108

Xhosa: *amagqirha* 41, 44, 48, 53; Cattle-Killing movement 46, 47, 51, 52; colonialism, cultural response to 46; cults of affliction 43, 44, 48; divination 43; Fitzgerald, response to 46–7; herbalists 43–4; *igqirha* 41, 43, 44, 47, 48, 53; medical syncretism 7, 48, 51, 55; medicine and colonial hegemony 41, 42, 45–6; Ninth Frontier War 53; prophets 46; traditional medicine 7, 43–5, 48; western medicine, disillusionment with 51, 52, 53; Western medicine, use of 41, 42, 48, 51, 55; witchcraft 43–4; *see also* Fitzgerald

Zaire: sleeping sickness, colonial treatment of 105
Zimbabwe: malaria, cultural responses to 10

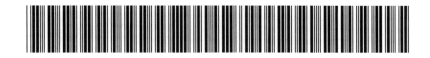